3 Months to
Your First 5K

3 Months to Your First 5K

5K

Dave Kuehls

A PERIGEE BOOK

A PERIGEE BOOK
Published by the Penguin Group
Penguin Group (USA) Inc.
375 Hudson Street, New York, New York 10014, USA

Penguin Group (Canada), 90 Eglinton Avenue East, Suite 700, Toronto, Ontario M4P 2Y3, Canada (a division of Pearson Penguin Canada Inc.)
Penguin Books Ltd., 80 Strand, London WC2R 0RL, England
Penguin Group Ireland, 25 St. Stephen's Green, Dublin 2, Ireland (a division of Penguin Books Ltd.)
Penguin Group (Australia), 250 Camberwell Road, Camberwell, Victoria 3124, Australia (a division of Pearson Australia Group Pty. Ltd.)
Penguin Books India Pvt. Ltd., 11 Community Centre, Panchsheel Park, New Delhi—110 017, India
Penguin Group (NZ), 67 Apollo Drive, Rosedale, North Shore 0745, Auckland, New Zealand (a division of Pearson New Zealand Ltd.)
Penguin Books (South Africa) (Pty.) Ltd., 24 Sturdee Avenue, Rosebank, Johannesburg 2196, South Africa

Penguin Books Ltd., Registered Offices: 80 Strand, London WC2R 0RL, England

While the author has made every effort to provide accurate telephone numbers and Internet addresses at the time of publication, neither the publisher nor the author assumes any responsibility for errors, or for changes that occur after publication. Further, the publisher does not have any control over and does not assume responsibility for author or third-party websites or their content.

First edition: July 2007

Library of Congress Cataloging-in-Publication Data

Kuehls, Dave.
    3 months to your first 5K / Dave Kuehls.—1st ed.
        p. cm
    ISBN 978-0-399-53402-7
    1. Running—Training.   I. Title.   II. Title: Three months to your first 5K.
    GV1061.5.K84 2007
    613.7'172—dc22

                                                    2007006160

PRINTED IN THE UNITED STATES OF AMERICA

10 9 8 7 6 5 4 3 2 1

PUBLISHER'S NOTE: Outdoor recreational activities are by their very nature potentially hazardous. All participants in such activities must assume the responsibility for their own actions and safety. If you have any health problems or medical conditions, consult your physician before undertaking any outdoor activities. The information contained in this guidebook cannot replace sound judgment and good decision making, which can help reduce risk exposure, nor does the scope of this book allow for disclosure of all the potential hazards and risks involved in such activities. Learn as much as possible about the outdoor recreational activities in which you participate, prepare for the unexpected, and be cautious. The reward will be a safer and more enjoyable experience.

Most Perigee books are available at special quantity discounts for bulk purchases for sales promotions, premiums, fund-raising, or educational use. Special books, or book excerpts, can also be created to fit specific needs. For details, write: Special Markets, Penguin Group (USA) Inc., 375 Hudson Street, New York, New York 10014.

Contents

PART 1   THE BIG QUESTIONS   1

1: Why Run? Why 3 Months? Why a 5K?   3

PART 2   WHAT YOU NEED TO KNOW
BEFORE YOU BEGIN   13

2: What to Wear   15

3: Where and When to Run   31

4: What to Eat   41

PART 3   TRAINING FOR YOUR 5K   49

5: How to Run   51

6: How to Stretch   63

7: Avoiding Injury   69

8: The Program   75

9: The Survivor Schedule   81

10: 34-Minute Time-Goal Schedule   87

11: 32-Minute Time-Goal Schedule   93

12: 30-Minute Time-Goal Schedule   99

13: 28-Minute Time-Goal Schedule   105

PART 4   YOUR FIRST 5K AND FUTURE RACES   111

14: The Race   113

15: What Next?   127

Resources   131

Index   133

3 Months to Your First 5K

THE BIG
QUESTIONS

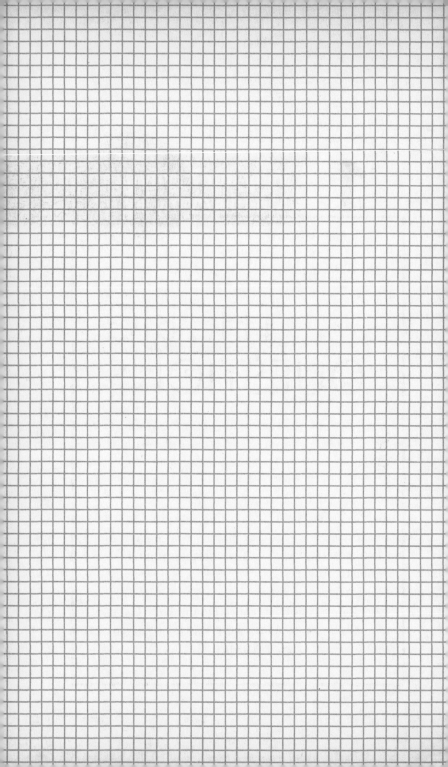

1 Why Run? Why 3 Months? Why a 5K?

YOU'VE SEEN THEM. On the sidewalks, as you are driving to work in the morning. In the park, as you are walking your dog in the afternoon. And in the evening, as you are gazing out from your front porch. They bounce by on residential streets, on trails, on walkways, their quiet conversations punctuated with laughter. They pull you away from your newspaper, draw you in toward them, as they disappear down the street, like a small parade that has passed you by.

Runners. They're everywhere now. Not just ticking off laps around the high-school track, puffing away on a treadmill at the local health club, or clicking a finishing time at the end of a jogging trail.

Runners are everywhere.

And that, admit it, has got you to thinking: Just how can I join them? You wouldn't have this book in your hand, open to the first page, if it hadn't.

Well, you've taken the first step by getting this book. Its aim is to be the most simple, basic running book out there, geared toward preparing the novice for the entry-level distance in the sport: 3.1 miles, or 5 kilometers, otherwise known as a 5K. Consider this book a hand that will reach out to you, helping you make that critical first step—commitment—and then guide you as you take more and more steps on your way to finishing your first race . . . to becoming a runner.

You like that phrase, don't you? *A runner*.

Okay, then. A question: What exactly is a runner?

Is it that super-thin, elite marathoner, who trains twice a day and logs 20 milers on a weekend?

Well . . . yes.

Or that ex–collegiate runner who trains seven days a week and wins road races weekend after weekend?

Well . . . yes, too.

Or how about that thirty-five-year-old mom who runs five or six days a week and races maybe ten times a year?

Affirmative.

Hey, but here's a secret: A runner is also—gulp—you.

Yes . . . you, an average Jane or Joe, maybe a few pounds overweight (or maybe more than a few pounds overweight), who has little or no athletic background, thinks sweating is something to avoid, and last wore gym socks in high-school P.E. class. Or maybe you love to play basketball on the weekends and you love working out in the gym, but you've never participated in an organized race before.

How, you may ask, can someone like you become someone like "that"?

WHY RUN?

Okay, you want to be a runner, but why? What, in addition to the status of being "one of the runners in town," can running do for you?

Glad you asked that question, because the answer is: a lot.

Running is good for you both physically and psychologically. Running helps you lose and control your weight. It is fun. Yes, fun. And entering 5K races that are geared toward raising money for worthy causes (like the American Heart Association or a local homeless shelter) is a good way to give back to the community.

Let's take these one at a time.

Your Physical Fitness

Running does a variety of things for you that will not only make running itself more enjoyable in the future, but that will benefit your overall everyday health in general.

Running lowers blood pressure. And helps control it. Exercise widens arteries, so blood flows through them more easily to deliver oxygen to working muscles. Wider blood vessels, less pressure.

Running strengthens the heart: A fit runner's heart actually beats fewer times per minute at rest, meaning there is less stress on an already stronger heart muscle.

Running strengthens the lungs: You breathe more deeply and fully, and it takes much more than a walk up the stairs to get you out of breath.

Running builds muscle: You will develop not only in the legs, but in the back and shoulders, the chest and arms . . . and the butt!

Running builds endurance: Gradually you can run farther. Also, everyday activities that used to wear you out no longer seem so taxing.

Running strengthens bones: Yes, it's true. Weight-bearing exercise causes bones to increase their density. The leg bones of seasoned runners are stronger later in life than those of people who have never run.

Running makes you tired, which makes you sleep more soundly. (Of course when you sleep, you may dream about running.)

Psych 101

Here's a little secret about running that runners often keep to themselves: 99 percent of the time, you feel better after going for a run than you did before. Is there any other activity that can do that for you? (Well, okay, I can think of one thing.)

Quite simply, running is a panacea, and those who run know all too well the withdrawal symptoms they go through when they can't run. Running fights a variety of bad things, while giving you a lot of good:

- **Running fights depression:** The blahs won't affect you as much.
- **Running fights anxiety:** What, me worry?
- **Running fights stress:** The less the better.
- **Running gives pep:** You'll get back that little spring in your step.
- **Running gives the slide-off effect:** Things that used to really bother you now "slide off" because of your run that day.

As you can see, running is like meditation, therapy, and a mini-vacation—all rolled in one.

How does it do all this? Well, when you've accomplished something like a half-hour run, you have a real reason to feel good about yourself. And feeling good about yourself leads to feeling good about many more things.

Weight Room

Running is also the best activity to do when you want to lose some pounds. It's better than walking, swimming, biking, basketball, weight lifting, or playing checkers. It burns more calories per minute than anything but cross-country skiing, which requires more equipment, skill acquisition, and snow than running does.

Also, once you take that weight off, running is the best way to keep from gaining those lost pounds again. After you've burned all those calories, your system metabolizes fat and you lose weight. And then when your body makeup contains less fat and more muscle, you have a higher resting metabolism (meaning you're burning more calories just walking around) because muscle burns more calories than fat does.

In short, running helps you lose weight and keep it off. Better than anything else.

Fun, Fun, Fun

It may not look like it to the cynical nonrunner, but a 3-, 4-, or 5-mile run (even a 10-mile run) can be a lot of fun.

The fun comes in three stages: before, during, and after the run.

1. **Before:** You'll be gearing up for your run hours or even a day or two ahead of time. Your body and mind get ready, and this focus is actually a positive, fun feeling to have. You anticipate what is to come in stage two.
2. **During:** The simple act of movement is pleasurable. Then there's the stress release. The lifting of the day's burdens. The social interaction if you're running with friends, and by all means, do run with friends. And, finally, that great moment when you know your run is complete—the last step before you slow to a walk.
3. **After:** That first refreshing swig of cold water or sports drink. A brief walk in the sun as you towel off. A little light stretching. That good feeling of "earned hunger," and the anticipation of a healthy meal that tastes great (just about everything tastes better when your hunger is real and comes from good hard work).

Running is fun in all of these ways and more. You just have to step out the door, put one foot in front of the other, and enjoy yourself.

Runners with a Cause

A vast majority of road races now give some or all of its profits to charity. Huge multicity events such as the Susan G. Komen Breast Cancer Foundation Race for the Cure series of 5K races (which included more than one hundred races and one million participants in 2005) offer you the opportunity to feel good in two ways. First, you're becoming a runner by training and racing the official distance (and getting all the nice benefits we've just mapped out), and second, you get the satisfaction of helping stamp out a major disease that needs to be cured soon. (Other races benefit homeless shelters, abandoned pets, and many more great causes.)

Running itself is simple, of course—we learn to do it instinctively, like walking or talking. But the sport of running requires technique, strategy, and a training plan, like other sports do. Most people wouldn't start ski racing or playing competitive tennis without taking some lessons first; consider this book your introductory course in the sport of road running.

And that brings up the two key questions for this book: Why three months? And why a 5K?

WHY THREE MONTHS?

THREE MONTHS. TWELVE weeks. Ninety days (give or take a day).

A season.

Put it this way: This book will take you at the beginning of summer or the beginning of fall or the beginning of winter (not recommended if you live in Point Barrow, Alaska) or the beginning of spring, and by season's end—voilà!—convert you into a runner.

As a duration, three months works because it's long enough to let you make changes (physically and mentally) from the running program, yet it's short enough so you don't give up along the way, thinking there's no end in sight. (Imagine if this book was titled *13 Months to Your First 5K*. How many of you would make it through a year of training without diving back to the couch, the remote, and a bag of tortilla chips for refuge?)

Three months also works because of a certain classically structured balance. Aristotle said all things must have a beginning, a middle, and an end. And so it is with this program. The beginning: one month to get your feet moving. The middle: one month to get your body to adapt. The end: one month to get you ready for the race.

To review: Three months is the perfect time frame to make you a runner because it's just enough time to whip you into shape (okay, *coax* you into shape) without trying your patience.

Other Things That Take Three Months

- walking across America
- a high-school football season
- a summer vacation
- potty training a puppy . . . I think

WHY A 5K?

WHAT EXACTLY WILL it take to get you to the finish line of a 5K?

Will it take a lot of overwhelming workouts? Runs so long that you collapse exhausted on the road? Weekly mileage that will give you blisters?

No and no and no.

That's the beauty of the 5K. You can train for it and still have a life. Sure, some workouts will be tougher than others. And you will run farther per day at the end of the program than you did at the beginning. And your weekly mileage will rise from single digits to low doubles.

But all of those things are gradual and doable, even for the complete beginner.

You simply have to lace up your shoes and follow the program in this book.

Other Things That Are 5K in Length

- just over twelve times around your high-school track
- twenty-four times down and back a football field
- that long walk to school
- the distance from the pub to your dorm room

WHAT YOU NEED TO KNOW BEFORE YOU BEGIN

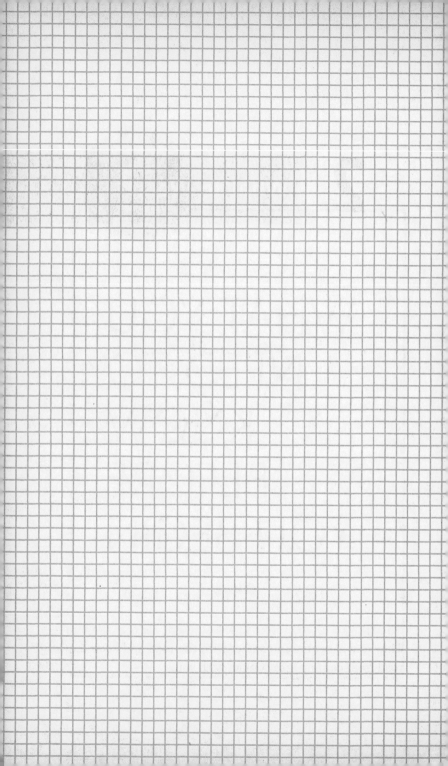

2   What to Wear

WHAT YOU HAVE on your feet, over your torso, and covering your legs can make a big difference in your enjoyment of the running experience. Bad shoes are like bad tires on your car: They can make you wobble or crash, causing injury. Bad shorts can chafe or bind. And a plain cotton T-shirt on a hot day will rub you the wrong way across the chest and underarms.

In short, wear the wrong things and you probably won't feel like running again. And that would mean you wouldn't finish this program.

Therefore don't skimp on your running gear.

SHOES

SHOES ARE *THE* key piece of equipment for any runner. They're what come in contact with the road and keep the road from coming into contact with you.

Imagine running down a concrete road—barefoot. How long before you'd break a bone in your foot? Bad shoes can lead to stress fractures—small hairline cracks in a bone—as well as to an assortment of other nagging foot problems, like blisters, black toenails, and "hot spots" on the tops of the feet from too much pressure there.

There are two keys to getting a good pair of shoes: cushioning and support. You should look for a pair that can give you both.

Most name-brand running shoes will provide you with enough protection for your run. Some shoes have more support (the "stability shoes" in each company's collection), some have more cushioning (they're cleverly categorized as "cushioning shoes"), and some have less of both so they can be as light as possible (these are usually known as "lightweight trainers" and are geared toward the highly competitive runner who is light of weight and foot). A good running-store employee should be able to help you pick the shoe that is just right for you, based on your height, weight, shoe size, running experience, gait, and foot plant (how your feet naturally hit the ground).

Buying Shoes

The Boulder Running Company is one of the premier running-shoe stores in the country. I visited and met with Mark Plaatjes, the marathon gold medalist at the 1993 World Championships. Plaatjes outlined the protocol of how he helps beginning runners find the right shoes:

1. He asks you to take off your shoes and socks.
2. He has you stand on one leg and bend that knee. While you do that, he's looking at the arch of your

foot to see whether it stays straight or flattens out. This will determine what kind of arch support you need in your shoes.

3. He has you stand up and checks your alignment— whether your knees and hips line up or whether they're bowed in or out.

4. He then asks you how much you run.

5. And where you run.

6. Finally, he puts you on a treadmill, videotapes your stride, and gives you what is called a gait analysis.

All of this helps him determine what running shoe is right for you.

Okay, so that's all well and good if you happen to have a great running-shoe store like the Boulder Running Company in your town. But what if you don't? What if your only option is a regular sporting-goods store? What do you do when you're facing a wall of eighty models of running shoes and the nearest employee is wearing a bowling shirt and flirting with the checkout girl?

First, grab three or four pairs of shoes in your size. Try each pair on.

1. Check the toe box—the area of the shoe that covers your toes. Here's a good rule of thumb: You should have a thumb's width between the end of your toes and the end of the inside of the shoe. Check both feet—they're usually not exactly the same size—and be sure to fit the bigger foot. If there's less room, your toes will be jammed up against the end of the shoe while you run (feet swell a bit when you're exercising), and not only is that rather uncomfortable, it can lead to black toenails (and ugly feet).

2. Check the heel cup or "counter." Like the toe box, the heel area should have some room (although much less) for movement during the up-and-down and side-to-side motion of running. If the shoe is too tight in the heel, you risk getting painful blisters on your Achilles tendon—a particularly annoying impediment to your running.

   How much wiggle room should you have inside the heel counter? You should be able to stick your little finger down the inside of the shoe all the way to the base of the heel.

   And while you're examining that part of the shoe, make sure that the heel counter is firm enough to support your foot when you're running. This is crucial to new runners who might be packing on some extra pounds; if that's you, a good running-store employee should steer you toward a stability shoe that's constructed firmly in this area. The counter should be stiff enough that you can't squeeze it flat, and it should retain its shape very well after you've tried.

3. Check the leather and laces (actually, few running shoes are made of leather, but "nylon and lace" isn't much of a pun): Make sure your foot can breathe in the shoe (always bring athletic socks or running socks when you try on new running shoes). And make sure that the laces, when they're tied securely across the top of the feet, don't bite into or rub across the tendons there.

4. Finally, once you have the shoes on—and make sure you put shoes on both feet—jog around the store for a bit. Rise up on the balls of your feet. Crouch down, too. (Specialty running-store employees will

often suggest that you run in them out on the sidewalk. Gary Muhrcke, the first winner of the New York City Marathon and now the owner of Super

Runners Shops in New York, insists that you run around the block in each pair you try on.) If you feel like you want to have them on your feet after you've tried them out thoroughly, there's only one thing left to do: Buy the darn things.

SOCK DRAWER

IN ADDITION TO carefully choosing your shoes, you should also take into consideration what socks to wear. (We're dwelling on the feet here, but for good reason: Your feet are the only parts of your body that hit the ground when you run.)

For running, cotton socks are out. "All they do is absorb sweat, get wet, bunch up, and cause blisters," says Plaatjes. "The synthetic blends are much better."

Once you've decided on synthetic-blend socks, there are really only two decisions you have to make after that:

1. **Thick sock or thin socks:** One provides more cushioning. The other leaves your feet feeling more "naked" in your shoes.
2. **How tight you want them.** Size-nine feet with size-ten socks will feel different than with size-eight socks, but both will work. It all depends on comfort and the feel you want when you're running.

WATCH OUT

ASIDE FROM YOUR shoes, a good sports watch might be the most crucial piece of equipment you'll need. A sports watch isn't just a stopwatch for timing yourself; it does two more things that are so important you might not think about them: First, it has an alarm function that wakes you up in the morning, so you don't miss your 6:30 a.m. run with Fido. And second, unlike a regular stopwatch, it still tells you the time of the day, so you don't miss that Wednesday group run at 5:30 p.m.

Sports watches come in many makes, models, and colors. Often you'll see two dozen or more on display. There are two main things to look for in a sports watch:

1. **The readability of the time.** This feature is crucial in the stopwatch mode. You should be able to read the digits clearly simply by turning your wrist at arm's length (sports-watch readouts come in a variety of sizes for different eyesights). You need this clarity because you'll be looking at the time while you're bouncing up and down as you run.

2. **The comfort of the watchband.** It should be tight enough that the watch doesn't turn around on your wrist while you're running, but loose enough that it doesn't bite into your wrist. Look for a watch with a band made of pliable rubber or a synthetic rubber, not a Velcro-like band, which will fray and rub after a while and will soak up sweat.

RUNNING BRA

As IMPORTANT AS it is to find a good pair of running shoes, it's just as important for women to find a good running bra. Since you'll be running longer distances on a frequent basis, you'll need a bra that's made for high-impact activities. The bra should be made from a breathable material and should fit snugly and comfortably, minimizing bouncing and holding the breast firmly in place.

THE FAIR-WEATHER BASICS:
SHORTS, SHIRTS, SUNGLASSES

AS WE'VE SAID, runners in this program might be carrying a few extra pounds. Some of those pounds might be congregating around the inner thighs. This can cause painful chafing if your shorts aren't long enough to cover your inner thighs. (You can also wear bike shorts–length half tights under your shorts; they'll cover your thighs and prevent the rubbing.)

Shorts that hang down to the knees and below might be all the rage in the NBA, but running in them will only cause problems when they get all wet from sweat and start to bag around the legs. (They also weigh about four times as much as a pair of running shorts.)

Cotton shirts are out, for much the same reason that cotton socks are out: Cotton absorbs sweat, and the shirt will hang like a dead weight around your shoulders. Instead pick shirts made of one of the new microfiber fabrics. These materials wick moisture away from your body, keeping you cool in the summer (and warm and dry in the winter, too).

Sunglasses are not a must, but if you have sensitive eyes, buy a pair that are light and wrap around the eyes. They should sit snugly, not bouncing as you run, but not tight enough to leave temporary dents in your head.

NOT ALL YOUR runs during this program will be done on sunny sixty-five-degree days. Depending when you start your three-month training cycle, you may also need gear for days when it rains or snows—or for days when the mercury in the thermometer tries to rise above the little glass tube it's in.

Rainy Days and Mondays

There are three main problems associated with running in the rain. Two are combatable and one isn't. The first problem is that you tend to get wet. But with the right kind of rain gear–a synthetic, rainproof shell jacket—your upper body can stay dry. A rain hat made of similar material can keep water off your head and your hair dry.

Which brings up the second problem: Rain can make it hard to see. Water drips into your eyes (or across your glasses or floats your contact lenses like boats), turning the crossing of a simple two-lane residential street into a potential disaster. What can you do? Well, a rain hat with a firm and long brim (this is the crucial element) can help keep most of the water out of your eyes, so you can see the minivan with the sixth-grade soccer team coming around the corner in time to get out of its way.

The third problem is not so easily controlled, and much of the enjoyment (yes, enjoyment) or discomfort of running in the rain will be associated with this: wet feet. Unless it's a light rain, which can be run in with minimal gear and minimal moisture collection by your shoes, running in the rain is sure to soak your shoes, socks, and feet, so that you land with that squishy sound. (Your wet shoes and socks will also begin to weigh more, too.) If you can't tolerate all this, your best bet when it's raining hard is to hit the treadmill at the local health club.

Here are a few pointers for running in the rain:

1. **Avoid grass.** It collects water like a sponge, and there's no quicker way to soak your shoes—aside from stepping in a deep puddle—than landing on a squishy stretch of sod.
2. **Don't step in those puddles.** Mom's advice holds true today. Watch for puddles during street crossings (especially near curbs, where water collects) and on trails that don't have efficient run off. When in doubt, step around rather than over, because once your shoes get wet, they won't dry out until after the run—way after.
3. **Wear thin socks.** They hold less water and dry more quickly.

Drying Your Shoes

JUST HOW DO you dry your rain-soaked shoes after a run? First off, loosen the laces, pull the tongues up, and pull out the insoles (most are removable). You can prop them against an outside wall to dry in the sun—if it has come out again, of course. Stuffing the shoes with crumpled-up newspaper speeds the process, as does setting them on or under a radiator if you have that kind of heating. A handheld hair dryer works well, too, if you're in a rush—and a clothes dryer will do the best job of all, but be prepared for some heavy-metal percussion coming from the laundry room.

Cold Comfort

Any run in temperatures below the mid-fifties calls for extra clothing and gear to complement the shoes, socks, shorts, and shirt you'd wear otherwise. That might just be a long-sleeved shirt instead of a short-sleeved one. Colder, and you can put a nylon shell over that. A hat, gloves, something to cover your legs (like running tights), and eventually, a thicker jacket, maybe made of Gore-Tex–type fiber that keeps you warm but also lets your skin breathe.

As with your shoes, you can get most of this cold-weather gear at a running store, and the employee there should know what you'll need. Some things you should keep in mind as you're shopping:

1. **The running hat:** The baseball-cap variety can keep your head warm into the low fifties, but for anything colder than that, you'll need a ski-cap style to lock in the heat and keep your ears warm, too. Make sure the cap fits snugly around your head, and—this is crucial—that it covers your ears with more than an inch of "fold space" at the bottom. This will make sure that the cap doesn't ride up over the ears while you are running, something that will most likely occur two miles into your run if you haven't bought the right-size cap.

2. **Long-sleeved shirt:** This works for temperatures in the mid-fifties and below (this will vary according to your cold tolerance; see page 26). Look for the same microfiber materials that you chose for your short-sleeved shirts. These will wick water away from your skin and help you stay warm. (You don't want a wet cotton long-sleeved shirt hanging off your arms during your run.)

Cold Tolerance

EACH OF US has a different comfort level when running in the cold. Some of us need to be bundled up like rangers on ski patrol when it's only in the high forties, while others can still run comfortably in shorts and a T-shirt in that weather. The trick is finding what's right for you—not for the next runner—and you'll only find out by running in the cold.

Still, there are a few basic pointers for all runners, no matter what their tolerance:

1. Know that your body in motion generates heat. Standing outside your car before you run on a cold morning, you will feel much colder than during your run (usually it takes about five minutes of running for your body's furnace to heat up). Therefore, keep in mind that the jacket that's keeping you warm and toasty while you're standing there will be like a heat lamp two miles into your run.

2. Overdress rather than underdress. Given what we have just gone over, this may seem like a contradiction, but dressing for a cold-weather run is a subtle art that will take practice to master. The key is not getting bone cold on your run, and this can happen if you don't wear enough clothes to cover your head, torso, hands, and legs. The simple rule is this: If you overdress, you can always take a layer off—a nylon shell (wrap it around your waist), a pair of gloves (tuck them into your waistband), or a ski cap (stick it in your jacket pocket). But if you underdress, you'll have no way to get warmer—and you might discover your mistake only when you turn for home and hit the windchill that you didn't feel on the way out.

3. **Nylon shell jacket and Gore-Tex jacket:** The lightweight shell is perfect for those in-between spring and fall days when the wind is blowing and temperatures can vary as much as ten degrees in and out of the wind and the sun. You can zip up tight, zip down to let more air in, or take it off on the run and tie it around your waist. Make sure the jacket has a good, reinforced zipper, because without it, the jacket won't be as versatile.

   On the other hand, a Gore-Tex jacket is too heavy to be tied around your waist. This kind of jacket should be worn only when you know the weather is cold enough that you'll really need it (again, you have to learn your personal cold tolerance). It is breathable, yes. But once you start running, it can get very warm inside.

4. **Gloves:** Like cotton running socks and vinyl records, cotton gloves are mostly a thing of the past (although they still have their champions). Modern running gloves made of synthetic materials fit better, last longer, and are warmer and more water resistant. Just make sure that the gloves aren't too tight. Your hands directly affect your overall running comfort. If gloves fit too snugly—believe it or not—that tension can easily be transmitted to the entire body, making the run a chore.

5. **Running tights:** They come in two styles: the looser-fitting stirrup kind that cover the legs like baseball pants and the tighter kind that stretch over your legs like a second skin (these are slightly warmer). The second kind come in thinner and thicker versions. The thick ones are for running when it's below twenty degrees out, although you

may want to think carefully before running in such conditions; it's doable if you can adapt and know what to wear.

Of course, you can do away with all of the above and spend the winter months on a treadmill. But you'll be missing out on one of the joys of running—a vigorous workout through the white stuff, when you can see your breath.

Hot Stuff

There are fewer options available for running in the heat than in the cold. Basically you can strip down the torso: For men, from a T-shirt to a singlet to bare chested; for women, from a T-shirt to a singlet to a jog bra. Each change is designed to put more skin, more surface area, open to the air, and therefore letting you cool off more efficiently (you'll need to apply extra sunscreen to those areas). Even a small thing, like thinner socks, can provide an extra cool comfort for the feet. But if you're running on a day when your feet are getting too hot in your shoes, you might want to consider taking that day off or running in the air-conditioned comfort of your health club.

Still, like running in the cold, there's something fun about a vigorous 4-mile run on a hot day, when the sweat pours off your head like a faucet and that first post-run chug of cold water feels like paradise.

Running in the Heat

Any run in weather above the mid-seventies should be handled differently than those nice, cooler runs. Make sure to dress light. Hydrate well before and after, and plan a stop by a water fountain during your route. It's a good idea to drink a sixteen-ounce bottle of an energy drink forty-five minutes before running in such temperatures. And another bottle when you finish. (For more on energy drinks, see chapter four.) Start slow, and don't worry if you sweat a lot. That's your body's way of staying cool. (The danger comes when you don't sweat enough or at all.) On hot days, you should also try to run early in the morning or late in the evening, when the air will be at its coolest.

3 | Where and When to Run

OKAY, YOU KNOW what you'll be wearing. How will you choose where you'll wear it? And when's the best time to get there? Like your choice of gear, these decisions will be based on various factors specific to each runner. This chapter will give you some help in narrowing down your own preferences.

WHERE TO RUN

The running surface you work out on can add to or detract from the run's effectiveness and your enjoyment. It can also help you avoid injuries—or help cause them. Different surfaces are better for different kinds of workouts: For instance, if you're trying to run at a faster pace, a track or well-tended trail is better than a hilly trail or a grass field, because you won't be slowed down by what you're running on.

Below is a list of several common running surfaces with their pluses and minuses, along with which kind of runs would be most appropriate in those settings.

Tracks: Recommended

Whether they're the new faster rubberized surfaces or the old cinder ones, tracks are the flattest, fastest, best-measured running surfaces you can find. (After all, running is what they're made for.) You'll often have plenty of other runners for company there, too. Tracks can often be found nearby, usually at high schools or colleges, within a short drive or maybe even walking (or running) distance. On a track, you know your exact distance; one lap is either 400 meters (most newer tracks) or 440 yards, which is one-quarter of a mile (most older tracks, usually dirt or cinders). Either way, it's not much of a difference—about nine feet. You won't be slowed down (or endangered) by car or bicycle traffic. There are no hills, sharp turns, or canted road angles, either. It's no coincidence that the world records at every distance have all been run on tracks. The minuses: Tracks can sometimes be crowded. And some people find it monotonous to go round and round the same course.

When you're on a track, you should usually be in the inside lane. (That's where you get the exact measurement.) However, if someone comes up behind you and says, "Track," she means that she wants to pass on the inside, and it's universal track etiquette to move out to your right and give the inside lane to the faster runner until she goes by.

Tracks are good for the repeat half-mile and 1-mile runs in this program. You'll get your best times there.

Trails: Highly Recommended

Whether a trail is made of dirt, cinder, or a mixture (trails paved with asphalt aren't really trails for our purposes; surfacewise, they're roads), running on one makes running a pleasure at virtually any time of day. Trails are usually located in city or national parks, and in these places, you'll probably see signs that make a distinction between *running* trails or paths and *hiking* paths. You don't want to run on the latter. Repeat: Hiking trails will end up being too rough and rocky, too twisty-turny, too steeply hilly, too full of foliage, or all of the above. They're basically an invitation to injury. For this program, stick to the running trails. They should be well marked by a trailhead sign or a sign near some sort of loop around an open field (a better running surface than simply grass; more on that later).

The biggest pluses of trails are that the surface is friendly to your feet, joints, and back, and that they're traffic-free and tend to be quiet. You're also likely to be able to find other runners there, so they're a good destination for a social run. Many trails are well marked for distance, often in half-mile or 1-mile increments. The minuses are that you may be a bit isolated at times. In the evenings or dark early mornings, especially if you're a woman, you'd be wise to run with a friend.

Overall, though, if you had to pick one place to do all of your training, a good running trail is almost certainly your best choice.

Roads: Not Recommended

Cement and asphalt roads should be avoided if at all possible. Country dirt roads can be good running surfaces, but you'll still have to deal with traffic, and these roads can be very rutted and bumpy. Well-traveled roads can be very dangerous: Cars can come from ahead or behind at any speed, and the drivers won't be expecting you. The air is often choked with exhaust. There really aren't any pluses associated with roads.

If you must run on roads, run with the cars coming toward you. Don't make the beginning-runner mistake of running in the same direction as the traffic; the cars will be coming up from behind you, and you'll have to trust every driver to see you and move out of the way, rather than vice versa.

Sidewalks: Not Recommended

Sidewalks are better than roads, only in that you don't have to worry about traffic—that is, until you come to a road. Sidewalks can also be unevenly paved and crowded. Many seasoned runners will often run on the grass right next to the sidewalk, but even that is a chore and can be dangerous, since you have to run looking both down at the surface and up to watch out for people ahead. Most sidewalks are cement, which is much harder than asphalt and can be damaging to your feet, joints, and back; there is no give, and most of the force of running goes back into your body.

Treadmills: Recommended

State-of-the-art treadmills with shock-absorbing suspension systems and runner-friendly rubberized surfaces are found nowadays in just about every health club and gym. You set the machine at a certain speed and then keep up with the moving belt. The sensation is slightly different than regular running; the debate rages over whether it's a little easier or a little harder. You'll have a control panel in front of you that can look like the captain's station on the starship *Enterprise;* don't be intimidated—most of it is unnecessary for simple running. (And for that really annoying guy who's ogling your running form, a phaser set on stun can be very useful.) The rails on either side of you make it easy to steady yourself or to step off if you want to, and there's a Stop button in front of you in case you need to quit running immediately.

Still, even with these precautions, treadmills can be tricky for the beginning runner. If you do decide to run on one, make sure you start at a walk to get used to the motion, start jogging at that same speed, and then accelerate very gradually. Be careful not to run up onto the non-moving front of the treadmill or to step off to the side of the moving belt—these are good ways to trip—and, perhaps obviously, don't slow down enough to be deposited on the ground behind the machine! The pluses: Treadmills are very precise. You'll know your exact distance and speed, which will give you confidence in your ability to run at a given pace. And the rubberized surface is also friendly to your joints.

Grass Fields: Recommended

Whether they're football or soccer fields, baseball diamonds, or open grass areas in recreational parks, grass fields can often be quiet, soft, safe, and pleasant places to run. The minuses are that grass can hide ruts beneath it, and fields aren't marked for distance. Still a grass field in the sun on a nice day can make for a nice break from the trail or the track.

THE TIME OF day when you run can be an important factor in your enjoyment of running, completing this program, and running your first 5K. If you're attempting this program in the heat of summer and you head out the door at three in the afternoon every day, you'll enjoy it less than if you head out later in the evening or early in the morning—simply because those times will be cooler.

Yet temperature is only one factor associated with running at different times of the day. Here is a brief discussion of the pros and cons of running at each time of the day.

Morning

If you run in the morning, you'll find that it's a great time for low temperatures and small crowds (sometimes: weekend mornings are the most crowded times on the running paths), and getting your run done first thing will energize you for the rest of your morning, maybe even your whole day. If you can get up early enough to run before work or school, mornings might be the best time to do all of your workouts in this program. You'll need to budget an hour for your running time so you won't be pressed, plus wake-up time before you get out the door (fifteen to thirty minutes), and then time after your run for a shower and breakfast before heading to work or school.

The major minus about running in the morning is for people who simply don't feel good enough at that time to go right out and exercise. Some people are meant to be sleeping at 5:30 a.m., not running hard miles on a track. If you're definitely not a morning person, you almost certainly already know it. But yet you might try a few morning runs on the weekends just to make sure. If getting out of bed seems like a real chore, please don't run in the morning. There is no quicker way to derail this program than setting that alarm clock at night, groaning in disgust when it goes off in the morning, and unplugging it and going back to sleep.

Late Morning

Running in the late morning is your second-best bet—if this fits into your schedule (it doesn't for most people). Late morning—say, 10:30 a.m. or so—can be a great time to train. You have a good night's sleep behind you. You have a good breakfast in the belly to fuel you. And that late-afternoon fatigue hasn't settled in. In other words, you're fresh, probably more fresh than you would be at 5:30 a.m., simply because you've given your body time to wake up. Some very good distance runners, like U.S. Olympic marathoner Steve Spence, have done their first runs of the day at midmorning, not early morning. Then again, running was Spence's job for many years, and he could fit in late-morning runs.

The only minuses might be a tendency to overeat at lunch following your run; eating a big meal after your run can weigh you down for the rest of the day. Yet there is a simple solution to this potential problem: Rather than have a big lunch, snack through the midafternoon. Eat two or three small snacks, like half a sandwich and an apple. Then some pretzels later. And then an energy bar at 2:30 p.m.

Lunchtime

Lunchtime is a very popular running time for business-people on the go who can't schedule early morning or evening runs because of kids or a commute or both. Lunchtime can be an efficient running option, but only if you can clear up certain things ahead of time:

1. **Are you allowed?** Some jobs don't give you the opportunity to run at lunch.
2. **If you are allowed, can you do it in the time allotted?** Can you get into your running clothes, out the door, through your workout, back to the workplace, showered and changed and fed, before it's time to be back on the job?
3. **Do lunchtime runs agree with you?** They could cause stomach distress before or after lunch (like late-morning runs, you need to snack often, not eat a big meal). They could energize you or do the opposite: put you to sleep at your desk. Only you will be able to tell how a 3-mile run at noon affects you. (Again, you might want to practice this during the weekend, so you don't end up in the bathroom all afternoon at work.)

Afternoon

For many, afternoon is the time that feels right for running. It is midday; the morning is over. If you can get out now, by all means do it—as long as it's not in the middle of a heat wave.

Afternoon runs offer more solitude than lunchtime or evening runs.

The drawbacks are the heat, and the feasibility. Most people are still at work at three in the afternoon!

Evening

Evening is the most popular running time, hands down. Running paths, roads, tracks, and treadmills are at their most crowded in this after-work period. Evening runs are a great way to wind down, releasing stress and getting you ready for a nice dinner and night. It's generally a bit cooler at this time of the day, too, simply because the sun has started to come down. Evening runs are great for running in groups or meeting a training partner (or somebody new).

The drawbacks are time constraints. Many of us have other commitments early in the evening; the key to a good evening run is the ability to manage those, so you can get to the path with time for your workout. Also, late in the fall and early in the spring, the sun sets early, and what can be a well-lit path when you start can be pitch-black when you finish.

Night

Running any time after the sun has gone down isn't recommended, unless you're running on a treadmill. Running outside at night is dangerous even for the seasoned runner. Small rocks and potholes in a road or path become like boulders and canyons at night. Dogs become more feral and protective of their territory. People might become more feral, too. Seriously, night really isn't a good time to be running outdoors at all.

4 What to Eat

SO WHAT DO you eat when you're on this running program? If you're new to running, you've probably heard that runners subsist on pasta, and you're ready to head to the noodle shelf of your grocery store and stock up. Then throw in a few energy bars, fill your refrigerator with sports drinks, and you've got all the nutrition you'll need to blast through your 5K at the end of three months, right?

Yes and no. While all those foods are runners' foods and they will help you to train and race better, if you tried to exist on them alone—or make them the major components of your diet—you'd fade out sooner rather than later, and we don't want you to fade out at all.

True, carbohydrates are what fuel your muscles when you run. But you need to eat a balanced diet, one that contains protein and some fat (yes, fat) if you want to fuel yourself as efficiently as possible.

LET'S LOOK AT what the following food components do (and don't do) for you, what foods are best, and how you can combine them all in a daily diet.

Carbohydrates

Carbohydrates provide muscles with glycogen, the fuel you burn when you run. Without it you would be running on fumes. When marathon runners "hit the wall," it's actually the point at which the runner has depleted his or her muscle glycogen reserves.

Good sources of carbohydrates are pastas, breads, and cereals. Whole grains provide more nutrients and are complex carbs, which burn slower and longer, and therefore are a more efficient fuel source than simple carbs, found in white bread, cookies, and sodas and other sugary drinks.

Protein

Proteins fuel muscle tissue and repair any damages to it. Without protein, your legs would eventually become too sore to run.

Good sources of protein are lean meats (including chicken and fish); dairy products like yogurt, milk, and cottage cheese; soy products including soy milk, edamame (soybeans), tofu (soybean curd), and tempeh (fermented soy "steaks"); just about any beans (garbanzos, butter beans, pinto beans, etc.); and nuts. Avoid fatty meats, especially the fast-food variety (which will not make you fast).

Fat

Fat balances blood sugar so your energy levels are consistent. It also can provide energy to burn when glycogen stores are low (though this probably won't happen during your 5K race or your training, unless you haven't eaten at all before a run).

Good sources of fat are fish, like salmon and tuna; olives; peanut butter and other nut butters; and healthy oils like olive, sunflower, and canola.

The Perfect Runner's Food

AS LONG AS you don't overdo it by spooning gobs of the stuff straight from the jar, peanut butter is a great food for runners because it supplies protein and the good kind of fat All-natural peanut butter, where you mix the oil from the top, is the best, though it's not as sweet and a bit harder to use.

YOUR BEST MEAL PLAN

EATING A GOOD balance of all three main types of foods—carbohydrates, proteins, and fats—is the key to good nutrition during this program. Rather than confuse you with numbers, I'll give you a good simple rule: Eat healthy carbs, a hand-sized helping of protein, and some fat during every meal, and snack twice a day (more on snacks below). Here is a sample daily meal plan that fulfills all of the above requirements:

Breakfast

- whole-grain cereal with low-fat milk (carbs and some protein)
- oat bagel with all-natural peanut butter (carbs and protein again, fulfilling protein and fat requirements)
- orange juice (carbs, water for hydration, and vitamin C)
- coffee (optional)

Lunch

- turkey sandwich on wheat bread with Swiss cheese, lettuce, and tomato (carbs, protein, fat)
- pretzels (carbs)
- lemonade (water, carbs)

Dinner

- angel-hair pasta with red sauce and a can of tuna (carbs and protein)
- tossed salad with light Italian dressing (some carbs, good fat)
- glass of red wine (optional)

In addition, you should drink six to eight eight-ounce glasses of water each day. This keeps your metabolism running smoothly and keeps you hydrated, which helps flush waste products out of the muscles, keeping stiffness and soreness at bay.

Snacks

The key to training for your first 5K is consistent nutrition, and that means three good meals a day. But equally important, and often overlooked, are the two to three between-meals snacks each day. Runners often tend to put all the emphasis on their meals and neglect to snack, which can eventually drive up hunger, causing you to overeat at meals. Or they simply reason that the healthy meals are all that count, and ruin their runner's diet with two jelly doughnuts at 10:30 a.m. and a jumbo candy bar at 3:30 p.m.

A good snack should be like a serving of protein—no bigger than hand sized. It should provide good carbs or some protein and fat.

Examples of good snacks include apples and other fruits (like peaches and tangerines), energy bars, and pretzels.

Examples of bad snacks include cookies, doughnuts, pastries, candy bars, sodas, and sugar straight out of the packet.

Energy Bars

Energy bars come in a variety of brands, flavors, and types. They are great ways to stock up on carbs, fat, and protein before you run and to put all those nutrients back into your body after your run. You should look for three things when choosing an energy bar:

1. **Taste:** If you don't like how it tastes, you won't want to eat it.
2. **Chewability:** Some bars tend to test your teeth and your jaw muscles. If you have the time for this, fine. If not, choose one with a little less elasticity.

3. Digestibility: You want to be able to run with the bar in your stomach, causing no discomfort or sudden detours to the bathroom.

Also energy bars can be used later in your running career, when you are going on longer runs and you want some energy on the way. Just cut them up into little pieces and store them in a small plastic bag. You can pop a piece into your mouth for energy at, say, the 7-mile mark of your 10-mile run.

Sports Drinks

Gatorade. POWERade. Accelerade. Ultra Fuel. There are more sports drinks out there than fingers on your hands. Generally they all contain water, some sort of simple sugar, and some potassium and sodium to replenish the amounts that you have lost while running. Sports drinks aid in recovery because they solve dehydration better than plain water (they're absorbed more quickly and more completely because of the sugar and potassium and sodium they contain). The sugar replaces expended glycogen, so they can fuel you before or during a workout.

That said, don't go overboard with sports drinks during the program. You don't need to guzzle a big bottle each day. Sports drinks should complement the other fluids you drink each day—like water, juice, and milk—not replace them. Think of sports drinks as your secret weapons in the fluid department. And like all secret weapons, their use shouldn't be too obvious.

Hint: If you've picked out your 5K race ahead of time, find out from the race organizers what sports drink they will offer during the race (there may be a fluid stop and there may not be). If they are going to offer a drink on the run, drink that one during the program to get used to the taste and feeling in your stomach.

Alcohol

Even the novice runner is aware of the connection between great runners—and many runners in general— and alcohol. Beer is the beverage of choice and running lore is filled with stories, true or apocryphal, about nine-teenth-century distance runners who took stimulating shots of whiskey during races (probably apocryphal) and about a certain Olympic marathon gold medalist who quaffed two beers the night before his victory (true). Alcohol has its pluses and minuses. Obviously, you don't want to overdo it—and the tendency with runners is to think they can overdo it because, "Hey, I just ran five miles"—but a beer or two after a good run can be one of the better feelings in the sport. Red wine has also been shown to have health benefits. If you tend to have a drink or two regularly, there's no need to quit. It will help you relax and sleep better and in that respect can actually aid in recovery.

But any alcohol can dehydrate you. And too much of it can cause liver damage and many other problems. Many veteran runners keep their alcohol intake on the low side in the weeks before a race. (And afterward that beer tastes even better.)

Be careful with hard liquor. Small amounts go a long way, and a runner's thirst is not something to let loose on a bottle of vodka or whiskey.

PART

3

TRAINING FOR YOUR 5K

5 | How to Run

SO NOW THAT you've gotten all the necessary equipment—a good pair of shoes, a trusty stopwatch, temperature-appropriate gear—and you know what to eat and where to train. What's next? Running!

FORM FOLLOWS FUNCTION

BEFORE WE GET to the actual schedules, now is a good time to talk about running form. All of you have probably taken a running stride or two before, even if it was just to catch a bus or escape the neighbors' dog. Here is a fact: Everyone's running stride is different, like snowflakes. Some people lift their knees higher than others do. Some carry their arms lower. Some land on the balls of their feet first and then hit their heels; some do it the other way around.

And you know what?

Any of these "quirks" in their running strides work for

them. (The quirks are actually, for the most part, compensations for individual differences, like weight distribution, leg length, torso alignment, and the like.)

That said, there are still some rules of the running road that apply to the technique of running, which we can all strive for.

Let's start from the top down:

Heads up. You'll want to run with your head as erect as possible so you don't put undue strain on your neck. (Here's a tip: Running form is all about efficiency—moving forward with as little wasted motion as possible—but it's also about relaxation. Forced form changes for the sake of running "perfectly" will likely add to tension. If it ain't broke, run with it.)

Eyes forward. Keep your gaze directed out and down, so you can see the ground.

Mouth open. Breathe through both your mouth and nose. Breathing through your nose alone won't give you enough air. You want to be as relaxed as possible when you run.

Lips loose. Lips are a key tension place. To see what we mean, open your mouth and breathe deeply with your lips clenched. Notice how your entire face, your neck, and even your chest area tense up? That tension is what beginning runners need to let go of throughout the body as they run.

Arms loose. Keep them relaxed, swinging freely from the shoulders, which are unhunched, to the elbows, which are at an unstiffened right angle, to the hands, which are closed lightly, like you're holding an egg in each palm.

Hands are another key tension point. Close your fists tightly and see what I mean. No one runs that way except bad actors on TV cop shows. Sprinters who are running 100 or 200 meters at absolutely top speed never clench their fists. Feel that tension up the forearms and into the biceps and shoulders? There's no way you can run one lap around a track like that, let alone a 5K. To have tension-free hands, keep the thumbs loose, not folded under the fingers. This helps the hands stay closed but loose, and the forearms, shoulders, and body tension free while running.

Shoulders straight. Don't pull them up, and don't try to run like you're at parade rest in the military. You want your shoulders square, but not so ramrod straight as to cause tension and not so leaned back that you throw your entire stride out of whack. A very slight forward roll of the shoulders keeps them relaxed and keeps you moving ahead smoothly.

Chest relaxed. Keep your chest muscles unengaged, not tight and expanded like you're posing in a body-building contest.

Hips aligned: Your pelvis should be aligned beneath the shoulders, tucked very slightly in, not out. Try walking with your rear end sticking out to see what we mean. Hip placement should be something your body does naturally while walking or running; the only problem occurs if you try to force a stride change to emulate someone—probably someone who's faster than you are. Remember that everyone's stride is different, and that for the most part, your body will find the stride that's right for you if you relax and let it happen.

A Word About Breathing

MANY BEGINNING RUNNERS think that an expanded chest is key to breathing well while running. After all, you want plenty of oxygen and what better way to get it than to breathe deeply? Well, the thought is good, but the execution is lousy. Expanding your chest does nothing but pump up your chest muscles when you breathe. To really fill your lungs with oxygen, you need to let your lungs inflate downward, not upward. This is called belly breathing because when you breathe that way, it's actually your belly that expands (moves out), not your chest.

Try this a few times to see what we mean. This is the breathing action you want to use during your running (though it won't be as forceful a breath as when you're sitting here concentrating on it). Eventually, with practice, this type of breathing will become second nature.

Knees forward, not up. Avoid exaggerated knee lift. Except when going up hills, the action with the knees should be more a forward swing than an up-and-down marching step. An exaggerated knee lift will just tire out your quadriceps muscles (the fronts of your thighs) as though you're running uphill, and you'll slow down when you don't have to.

Ankles loose. Your ankles should stay limber and relaxed; they should feel like fulcrums from which your feet hang. Tight ankles—try tensing them up now to see how they feel—will slow you down more effectively than running through molasses.

Feet relaxed. Keep your toes and arches loose. A lack of tension is the first key to a solid foot strike. The second is to land near the back of the ball of the foot. Anything farther forward and you start to get up on your toes, which causes (you guessed it) tension; if you land on the very back of your heels with your feet flexed, your weight will shift backward and fight your forward momentum. Foot strike is a tricky thing. Again, your body will lead you to how it wants to run. Generally you should follow your body's lead.

YOUR FIRST STEPS

THE FIRST STEPS you take as a runner will be—and this is not hyperbole—monumental. If you are serious about this book—training and racing a 5K and becoming a runner—then what you do with those first strides—the wonderful moment when both feet are off the ground at the same time, floating—is crucial. Those steps won't just lead you three months down the road to the finish line of a 5K; they'll lead you—whether it's three months, three years, or thirty years down the road—to a running lifestyle that is full of fitness, fun, and accomplishment.

Okay, so you've got your shoes and shorts and shirt. You're on a running path at a local park (wait till that group passes) or the high-school track or a country road (not too bumpy). You know what makes for good running form.

Now, here's what you do. Reach out with your dominant hand. For example, if you're right-handed, gently close that hand and hold it in front of you.

Now, eyes level, looking ahead. Always ahead.

Take a deep breath.

Exhale and swing your extended arm back.

At the same time, lift the knee on that side and swing the opposite arm forward.

Let your arms swing like that, alternating, and let them be the impetus that picks up your knees.

As a knee comes up, push off a bit with your other foot.

Leave the ground.

You have just taken your first step toward becoming a runner.

Congratulations.

THE PRIDE OF GOING FARTHER

ONCE YOU TAKE those first steps and cover that initial distance (this program starts with a half-mile run, roughly five minutes of running), you'll want to go farther. It's only natural to want to test yourself, as long as you gradually build those longer runs into your schedule—and that's what this schedule outlines.

And with more steps and more distance—as that half-mile becomes 1 mile and that mile becomes a mile and a half and that becomes 2 miles—comes a certain pride. We'll call it the Pride of Going Farther.

At first it is pride in how far you can go in one run without stopping. Then you'll find motivational pride in logging more runs of a certain distance per week, say three 4-mile runs, instead of two. You'll start to get interested in your weekly mileage, and you'll push it up from, say, 10 to 15. And then to 20.

Lifestyle Plus

THE RUNNING LIFESTYLE: You've heard this phrase or will hear it sometime soon after starting this program. It is something that encompasses all of the above—the training, the dress, the nutrition, and more. Something intangible, yet definitely there. It includes how you wake up in the morning, more refreshed and ready to meet the day. And how you tackle the morning, with a spring in your step or a relaxed mojo in your mind (especially if you've already gone for a run). How you manage the afternoon, with more energy than before and less of a need to take a nap (though naps can be important). It will also affect your evening meals, which will be healthier, and therefore you'll be more alert at night to read a good book or watch a classic movie. You'll get to sleep more quickly and sleep more soundly. And when you sleep, you will often dream of running.

THE TRAINING ELEMENTS

THIS TRAINING PROGRAM utilizes three different types of run: the endurance run, the strength run (often called speedwork), and the recovery run. Each week you will be including at least two of the elements, eventually three. Toward the end of the schedule a fourth run will be used to prepare you for the race experience. We will call this special run the Starting-Gun Strider.

Log On

KEEPING A RUNNING logbook is a great way to track your running progress. Writing in 3 for three miles on Monday, or 4 for four miles on Wednesday, or 3 x ½ for three times running a half-mile on Friday, and then looking back on your progress, is a great boost for your next session. Putting something down on paper makes it permanent, "in the books," something you can look back on (and congratulate yourself for) days or weeks or months down the line.

Logbooks help you see where you're going. And know where you've been. There are several kinds to choose from in the bookstores, from ring-binder diaries with room for your workouts ("an easy 3 miles"), the day's weather ("raining cats and dogs, but I ran anyway!"), and personal thoughts about your workout ("felt sluggish at first but at the end I was pumped") to simple running calendars, with a small square below each date where you can record your mileage.

Personally I prefer both. The ring binder is great because of all the information you can pack into it. The calendar is great because, instead of just one or two days open in front of you, you can see a whole week's or month's workouts in their entirety.

Looking at the calendar is like having a full map of a state in front of you; the ring-binder diary is like having individual maps of each county you cross on your journey. It's up to you whether you want one, the other, or both.

The Endurance Run

The goal of an Endurance Run is simply to cover a distance without stopping or walking. (This is a running program and your goal is to run, not walk, these workouts and the whole race.) The actual distance is relative to where you are in the training program. At first it's just a half-mile. Then 1 mile. Then two, three, working up to 4 or 5 miles by the end of the three months. These runs will be done at a slow, easy pace, the goal being simply to finish the workout.

The Walks

ALTHOUGH YOU WON'T want to walk during your 5K or on any of your endurance runs, you will see from the schedules that walking plays an important part in each run. Walking is used to warm up the muscles, circulatory system, and respiratory system for your run; and it is used to cool down the same after you finish. Walking also helps to build endurance. So make sure to keep to your walking schedule as well as your running schedule.

In this program, walks are done at a conversational pace. Start easy and then work up to a pace where you're breathing a little hard, but not so hard that you can't hold a conversation with someone. Wear your running shoes and attire, and at the end of your warm-up jog, simply take a few moments and stretch and/or take a few deep breaths, and then begin your run for that day. At the end of your run, transition to the walk after a few moments, but save the stretching, if you want to do some, for after the walk.

So what is this "endurance" that these runs give you? It's the ability of the body to keep going for an extended period of time. Each Endurance Run actually prepares the body, physically and mentally, to go farther the next time out—presuming you give the body time to rest a few days—and grow stronger from your Endurance Run. That is, you wouldn't do an Endurance Run on Monday night and then another one on Tuesday morning expecting to suddenly be fitter. The body doesn't adapt quite that fast.

The Strength Run

The goal of a Strength Run is to push the body slightly, to enter a zone where you know you're really working, and then to hold it for a certain time or distance—four minutes, maybe, or a half-mile. Strength Runs will be shorter overall than the Endurance Run, but you'll do them at a faster pace or on a tougher surface (uphill, for example). These runs will be worked into your running program during the second month, after you have enough endurance and fitness to recover from them.

The function of this run is to develop strength or stamina, the ability to keep running at a certain pace when you feel uncomfortable and want to slow down.

The Recovery Run

Shorter than the Endurance Run and slower than the Strength Run, the Recovery Run is the key workout in this program. Without it, a running program would wear you down and you'd quit running and go back to bowling or lawn darts. The Recovery Run lets your body recover from the other, harder workouts. The Endurance and Strength

Runs stress the body in ways that cause a positive, fitness-enhancing response—if you give your body time to put those workouts to use. Continual stress without recovery will cause the body to break down.

The function of a Recovery Run is to teach your body to recover while still running. This is a talent that all true runners cultivate and nurture. Without it, they would not still be running.

The Starting-Gun Strider

There you are, lost among several hundred or even several thousand runners at the starting line of your first race. You've done your warm-up jog and stretched a bit. Butterflies flutter in your stomach. The starter gives the runners their commands.

The gun goes off. It's like chaos in a crowded theater. Suddenly you're running in an environment you have never, ever encountered in practice. What do you do? Run sideways? Back up? Dog-paddle?

The goal of the Starting-Gun Strider is to give you confidence when the gun (or air horn or whistle) sounds—a crucial moment that can either sap your strength or help position you for a successful race. With a Starting-Gun Strider, the key is to develop an easy, relaxed pace. Since you'll be using this type of run at the beginning of the race, practice by starting slowly with your arms out to guard against being bumped and knocked off balance.

This run will teach you how to get going amid a crowd without losing any adrenaline, confidence, or endurance.

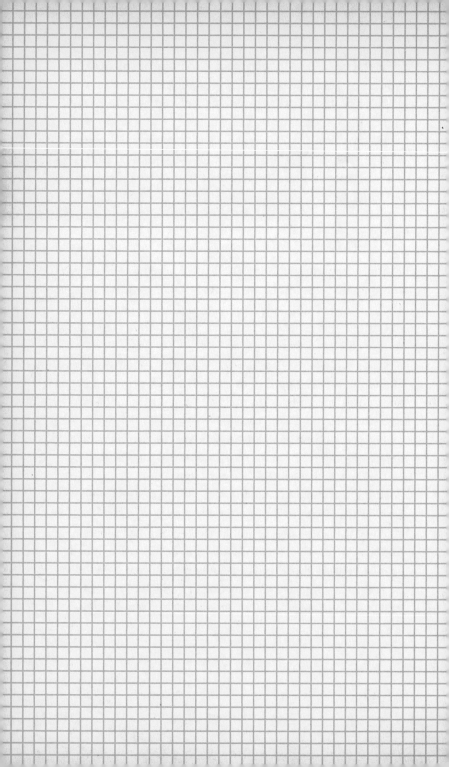

6 How to Stretch

TWO OR THREE times a week, you should spend twenty minutes on some basic stretches. This stretching will help you in a variety of ways:

1. It will help lengthen your stride and therefore make running at a given pace easier.
2. It will help prevent running injuries to both the muscles and joints.
3. It will make you feel better. Following a run, there is less stiffness and soreness in stretched muscles than in tight, bunched muscles.

So when should you stretch? The best time is just after an easy workout, when you are not feeling worn out and fatigued. Don't stretch when your legs are feeling sore; it can feel good, but it can also cause more problems by overstressing muscle fibers that are already slightly damaged, leading to prolonged recovery time.

A common mistake is to stretch before running as a warmup. The problem with this is that "warming up" isn't a figurative term; it really means to become warmer, and stretching doesn't generate heat. The best way to warm up is to start walking and then jogging. Stretching cold muscles won't make them more flexible, just more uncomfortable—and you could strain them that way, too. A muscle's flexibility is increased if it's stretched when it's already warm and loose from being used for a while—like after a run.

When you begin, hold your stretches for five to ten seconds. When you're several weeks into your stretching program, you can hold your stretches for about twenty seconds. Stretch the muscle until you feel a gentle but firm lengthening sensation—*not* pain—and hold that position for those few seconds, then release it, and repeat the procedure once or twice.

THE THREE BASIC STRETCHES

DOING THESE THREE basic stretches two to three times each week should help most runners increase their flexibility.

The Calf Stretch

Your calf muscles (technically, the gastrocnemius) are the muscles that run down the backs of your legs from your knees to your heels They're responsible for extending your feet, like you do when you push off the ground while running or walking.

For this stretch, stand close to a wall with both palms flat against the wall. Place the toes of one foot about six inches away from the wall. Bend that knee slightly. Place the other foot on the ground, about two feet behind the first one. Press your hands against the wall and lean forward toward it, feeling a pleasant stretching sensation from the back of your knee to your heel. Hold it, and release. Then repeat on the other side.

The Quadriceps Stretch

Your quadriceps, or "quads," are the large muscles that run down the fronts of your thighs from the hip to the knee. As you might guess from the name, there are four of them in each leg. Their primary function is to straighten your leg at the knee, as a runner does when she pushes forward off her back leg, or as a cyclist does to push down on the pedals. (Ever notice good cyclists' extremely large, muscular quads? Don't worry—runners' quads don't get that big, but they do get muscular and strong.)

For this stretch (starting with the left quads), stand on your right foot, steadying yourself with your right hand against a wall or chair back (or anything firm). With your left hand, reach down and cup the front of your left ankle, then bring the left foot up behind you toward your butt. Stand tall and feel the stretch down the front of your left thigh. Hold it and release. Repeat with the other leg.

The Hamstring Stretch

The hamstrings, or "hams," are the muscles that run down the back of your legs (three on each leg) from the hip to the knee. They're responsible for bending your knees, and they also work to move your whole leg back from your torso. Tight hamstrings can lead to all sorts of problems, whereas loose hamstrings will help make running easy and efficient.

For this stretch, find a chair or bench and place one heel on it, keeping your leg as straight as you can, while standing tall on the other leg. Lean forward gently over the leg that's out in front of you and feel the stretch along the back of your leg (you might feel it in your calf, too). Hold it, and release, stretching carefully but fully. Repeat with the other leg.

ADDITIONAL STRETCHES

IN ADDITION TO the basic stretches, there are other stretches you can try to increase both your flexibility and mobility.

Lower Back Stretch

Lie on your back with your legs straight. Bend one leg and pull that knee up toward your chest with both hands (this will also stretch the gluteal—butt—muscles and upper hamstrings). Hold and release. Repeat with the other leg.

Soleus Stretch

Your soleus muscle runs between the calf and the Achilles tendon at the back of each leg. It's only partly visible because it's beneath the other calf muscles, but it's essential to running.

Stand with both feet close to a wall (or something else); use your hands for balance and squat down, placing most of your weight on one leg. Feel the stretch in your lower leg, just above your ankle. Hold and release, and repeat with the other leg.

Total Back Stretch

You will need a pull-up bar for this. Simply grab the bar with both hands and gently hang from it. Feel the stretch in your lower and upper back.

Iliotibial (IT) Band Stretch

The IT band (pronounce each letter: *eye-tee band*) is a common name for a muscle called the tensor fascia lata, which runs down the outside of your leg from your hip to your knee. It helps to control and stabilize your leg while you move forward. Using it a lot can make it *too* tense, which, like most other tension, is bad for your running career.

Stand with your right side about two feet from a wall, then cross your left leg in front of your right. With your right hand on the wall, let your right hip sway in toward the wall. Feel the stretch along the outside of your right thigh. Hold and release, and repeat on the other side.

7 Avoiding Injury

THE GOAL OF this book is twofold: To get you to the finish line of a 5K in your desired time (or simply to finish it, if you choose the Survivor program) and to keep you running after that race. Neither of these goals can be accomplished if you are injured.

So how do you prevent running injuries?

INJURY-PREVENTION TIPS

ALWAYS BE GRADUAL in your buildup. Don't jump into a hard run right off the bat or leap up in mileage from one day or week to the next. Muscles and joints have to be prepared for increased use and extra exertion. By following this program, in contrast, you will increase your mileage from day to day and during the week only in very small increments, thereby working to stay injury-free.

Stretch: There are several basic stretches you can perform two to three days a week to keep injuries from occurring; a loose, stretched muscle is less likely to pull or tear than a tight, unstretched muscle. See chapter six for more details.

Ice: It might take a little getting used to, but icing down your leg muscles is a great way to recover from a hard a run like your half-mile or 1-mile repeats and to prevent injuries. The cold from the ice stops the progress of the microscopic tears in muscle fiber, which you experience as soreness, and it also aids in the elimination of waste products like lactic acid that can exacerbate the soreness and tightness.

The best way to ice a muscle is by using an ice cup. Simply fill a Dixie Cup with water and then freeze it. When you're done with a run, use the ice cup by holding the paper cup and rubbing the ice over the muscle. As the ice melts, peel back the paper of the cup. It's best to ice an area for five to eight minutes, not just five seconds or so!

Another method is the cold shower or bath. If you can stand it, run cold water over your legs following your run or slip your legs into a cold bath. (Getting into a cool bath and gradually adding cold water will lessen the shock.)

Wear the right shoes: Shoes that don't fit, have poor cushioning, and/or are old and worn out are invitations to injuries. Follow the advice in chapter two on getting a great pair of shoes and you can put a check mark next to this injury-prevention tip.

Run on forgiving surfaces: Trails, fields, and tread-mills should be the places where you're doing most, if not all, of your running. Avoid roads and cement side-walks to decrease the damage from pounding your feet and legs on those surfaces.

Watch downhills: Downhill grades on trails put more stress on your ankles and knees. Slow down on down-hills or try to avoid them altogether during runs. (To slow down while running downhill, simply concen-trate on shortening and slowing your stride and keep-ing your back perpendicular to a hypothetical flat surface; don't lean forward or back.)

HOW TO DEAL WITH INJURIES

Now THAT YOU know how to prevent injuries you should be fine. Still, some injuries might occur. Here is a list of the likely injuries that beginning runners might encounter and some advice for how to deal with them:

Muscle strains: Calf, quadriceps, and hamstring strains can occur when you make a jump from walk-ing to running. It will feel like a concentrated numb or sore spot in the muscle, but it's really no cause for major concern. Simply ice it and run easy for the next day or two, and the strain should go away. Then make sure to stretch that muscle regularly.

Hot spots: Hot spots occur on the bottom of the foot, often near the small bones below the toes (the metatarsus). They feel sore to the touch and often flare up during a run only to go away when you are walking afterward—or vice versa. If you experience a hot spot, ice the painful area. Make sure your shoes are cushioned enough and that you're running on soft surfaces. (Hot spots can morph into something much more serious called a stress fracture—a hairline crack in a bone. If this happens, you'll know it right away, because your foot will be too painful to walk or run on at all.)

Runner's knee (chondromalacia patellae): Perhaps the most common malady among beginning runners, this knee pain is a general throbbing you'll feel after a run and can simply be the knee's reaction to beginning a running program. It can also be a warning that there is too much stress on the knee and that you should check your shoes and running surfaces, ice your knees, and stretch your quadriceps more to loosen up those major muscles and put less stress on your knees when you are running. A great preventive measure is to strengthen the quads with a simple weightlifting exercise called leg extensions: Sitting with your legs straight out, your knees supported and your lower legs hanging off the chair or bench, slowly lower and raise your lower legs while lifting a light-to-moderate weight at your ankles. Wraparound ankle weights are ideal, but a couple of big books will work, too—and all gyms have leg-extension machines. Do three sets of ten slow repetitions, about two or three times per week with a day or more off in between.

Black toenails: If your shoes are too small (or your socks are too thick) and your toenails constantly hit the front of the shoe, you might get black toenails.

Normally the big toe's nail is the first to turn black, but other toenails can change color also. Once a toenail turns black, you either have to wait until it eventually falls off or get it surgically removed by a podiatrist. Black toenails have a simple solution: new shoes or thinner socks. Make sure to check the toe box of the shoes when you buy them, pressing a thumb down at the tip of your big toe. If the toe reaches the end of the shoe, the shoes are too small.

Sore Achilles tendon: This problem is at the opposite end of the foot and shoe. Sometimes the shoe's heel counter is too stiff or tight, and this can lead to rubbing on your Achilles tendon, which in turn can lead to blisters and rubbed-off layers of skin. This problem can be very painful, but it isn't serious. First, you need to attend to your heel. Make sure the wound is clean by washing it well. While you're waiting for it to heal, always wear a clean pair of socks. If the abrasion is severe, cover it with a bandage. Next, get to the root of the problem. You either need to soften up your heel counters by bending and twisting them or get another pair of running shoes. (Future problems can be prevented by checking the heel counters before you buy shoes.)

Shin splints: These are pains along the fronts of the shins that usually occur when you first start a running program or move into faster-paced running. Shin splints, when severe, are so painful that you can't run with them. It feels like someone has scraped the skin and bone off your shins with a power sander. The immediate treatment for shin splints is to ice your shin(s). Later you should work into a stretching program for the calves. Then you'll want to strengthen the muscles in the fronts of your shins—the tibialis anteriors—with some toe raises: Sit in a chair with your feet out in front of you and your knees flexed. Pull your toes toward you and feel the shin-area muscles working.

Sciatica: This injury is literally a pain in the butt. It can also radiate down the back of your thigh. It's due to a tightening of a small gluteal muscle called the piriformis, which can press on the sciatic nerve and pinch it a bit. To alleviate this pain, loosen the gluteal muscles around the nerve to give it some room. This can be done by massaging the muscles, putting hot packs on them, using hot balm and rubs, and/or stretching the area. A good stretch is to lie on your back, cross your legs at the knees with the painful leg on top, and gently pull the other knee with both hands to bring the fronts of your thighs toward your chest. You should feel a slightly more pleasant pain in the butt.

IT band strain: This is a micro tearing of the IT band that feels similar to shin splints but goes down the outside of your thigh. To alleviate it, ice the area, stretch the other major leg muscles, and, when ready, gently stretch the IT Band (see page 67).

8 The Program

IN THE FOLLOWING chapters, we finally get down to the nitty-gritty of the program—spelling it out for you day by day, week by week, and month by month. It is not written in stone. There will be days when you might have to miss a workout (but try to make it up later) or modify it because of time constraints, fatigue, or both. The important thing is to try to stay as close to the schedule you've chosen as possible. Consistency is the key in this program—or any other training program, for that matter. As long as you keep doing the workouts, progressing through more distance and more demanding strength runs, mixing in the recovery runs, and resting well, you should make it to the starting line of your first 5K in top shape.

And then all you have to do is one simple thing: Run it!

THE SCHEDULES

WHAT FOLLOW ARE several training schedules for running your first 5K. First off is the basic finisher or Survivor schedule. This should be used by anyone who's brand-new to the running experience. Your goal with this schedule is simply to finish the race without walking. It contains fewer taxing runs than the other schedules, less overall mileage, and a generally less strenuous and more beginner-friendly approach to a running lifestyle.

Training Motivation

THERE WILL BE moments during your training—and periods of time that are longer than moments—when you experience doubt about your running: *Can I do this workout? How do they expect me to run four days a week for three whole months? Will I ever get the heck to the finish line?*

Don't worry. These doubts are normal, and they usually go away after the first flush of a workout—that trickle of sweat down the forehead, when you become focused on the task at hand.

If the doubts don't go away, remember all the benefits you'll receive from a regimen of healthy running:

- You'll wake earlier in the day, with more energy.
- Work, school, or both will seem easier to a degree. Running energizes the brain by stimulating the production of sense-sharpening and mental focus—enhancing endorphins. It also helps you cut down on stress—so that history

test or coworker who never cleans out the coffeemaker doesn't cause you as much anxiety.

- You'll have more hunger, but you'll eat more healthily. (After a while, you'll drive by your favorite fast-food place without even considering pulling in.) As you get fitter and leaner, you'll feel too good about your body to load it up with junk.
- You'll have more friends. Running is a great way to meet—and keep—new friends. In fact, people who meet in races and run them together often become lifelong friends—let's call them fast friends—because they now share a bond: what they endured together and accomplished together.
- You'll have more fun. Because you'll have more energy and more friends, of course, and because . . .
- You'll look better. Losing weight, gaining muscle tone, and getting that glow on your face all add up to a more physically attractive you.
- Your dog and in-laws will love you more. (Okay, maybe just the dogs, because they'll get to go on longer outings.)

Next are the time-goal schedules. These are geared toward the beginning runner who wants a specific time goal to shoot for when starting off down the twelve-week road to that first 5K. These schedules all start with a month of basic training that's designed to get you up to more than two miles of running at one time. After that period, each schedule kicks into its own time frame. The goal times: thirty-four, thirty-two, thirty, and twenty-eight minutes. Your actual race may be faster or slower, and you'll probably end up between two of these times. Don't worry yet about which of the four you should choose; let the first month be your guide. After that point, those 5K times will be more than just a list of numbers.

Each time-goal schedule is structured basically the same way: in three blocks of one month each, with the goal of each block/each month, spelled out accordingly.

MONTH ONE: First steps, work on building endurance and incorporating rest and recovery. The goal is to start running and gradually work up to running more—without getting injured, overly fatigued, or sick and tired of running already!

MONTH TWO: More endurance and now some strength. You're still making rest and recovery a priority. The goal is to become able to run farther and be a stronger runner. You should feel your confidence in running blooming. Also, at the end of the month, another feeling should be emerging: anticipation.

Your first 5K is only a month away.

MONTH THREE: More endurance and strength, plus two weeks before the race. Endurance, strength, and confidence should be peaking. You're still resting and recovering on key days, but those days feel much lighter than before. You are getting fit.

THE LAST WEEK: Each schedule has a special last-week, race-ready schedule, unique to itself, but with a logical approach that builds upon your training. That's because in the last week your goal is not to continue to train vigorously, but to step back a bit and get race ready for the big day at the end of your three months.

Schedule Symbology

Here is a translation of a typical workout with the abbreviations used in the schedules that follow:

$$3 \times \tfrac{1}{2} @ 5:10$$

Translation: three times a half-mile at five minutes and ten seconds.

More thoroughly: After your warm-up, do three half-mile runs with rests between them,* and try to run each of the three half-miles in about five minutes and ten seconds.

When Illness Interrupts Your Schedule

GENERALLY, A COLD, a sore throat, and/or cough is a sign you should take a few days off from your training program. You can run through a mild cold, although it's not advised— if you keep training when you have a cold, you can end up more sick than when you started. If you have a fever and your body aches, be sure to take at least three or more days off.

When you're feeling better again, ease yourself back into your training program. Depending on how long you were out, you may want to backtrack a bit, or you may pick up where you left off. Whatever you decide, do what's best for your body, paying attention to any excessive exhaustion as a sign you may be pushing yourself too hard.

---

* Throughout all the schedules, the rest periods between fast runs on Strength Run days should be very easy jogging for (a) about the same amount of time that the fast run was prescribed at (5:10 in the case above), or (b) half the distance of the fast run (a quarter mile in the above case), whichever's more convenient. (If you were to run the workout above on a track, for example, jogging a slow lap for a quarter mile would be very convenient.)

The Survivor Schedule: Finishing the Race

THE FIRST MONTH

WEEK ONE

MON: walk ½ mile to warm up; run ½ mile;
walk ½ mile to cool down

TUES: rest and recover

WED: walk ½ mile to warm up; run ½ mile;
walk ½ mile to cool down

THURS: rest and recover

FRI: walk ½ mile to warm up; run ½ mile;
walk ½ mile to cool down

SAT: walk ½ mile to warm up; run ¾ mile;
walk ½ mile to cool down

SUN: rest and recover

WEEK TWO

MON: walk ½ mile to warm up; run ¾ mile;
walk ½ mile to cool down

TUES: rest and recover

WED: walk ½ mile to warm up; run 1 mile; walk ½ mile to cool down

THURS: rest and recover

FRI: walk ½ mile to warm up; run 1 mile; walk ½ mile to cool down

SAT: walk ½ mile to warm up; run 1¾ miles; walk ½ mile to cool down

SUN: rest and recover

WEEK THREE

MON: walk ½ mile to warm up; run 1¾ miles; ½ mile to cool down

TUES: rest and recover

WED: walk ½ mile to warm up; run 1¾ miles; ½ mile to cool down

THURS: rest and recover

FRI: walk ½ mile to warm up; run 1¾ miles; ½ mile to cool down

SAT: walk ½ mile to warm up; run 2 miles; ½ mile to cool down

SUN: rest and recover

WEEK FOUR

MON: ½ mile walk ; 2 mile run; ½ mile walk

TUES: rest and recover

WED: ½ mile walk; 2 mile run; ½ mile walk

THURS: rest and recover

FRI: ½ mile walk; 2 mile run; ½ mile walk

SAT: ½ mile walk; 2¼ mile run; ½ mile walk

SUN: rest and recover

THE SECOND MONTH

WEEK FIVE

MON:	½ mile walk; 2¼ mile run; ½ mile walk
TUES:	rest and recover
WED:	½ mile walk; 2¼ mile run; ½ mile walk
THURS:	rest and recover
FRI:	½ mile walk; 2¼ mile run; ½ mile walk
SAT:	½ mile walk; 2½ mile run; ½ mile walk
SUN:	rest and recover

WEEK SIX

MON:	½ mile walk; 2½ mile run; ½ mile walk
TUES:	rest and recover
WED:	½ mile walk; 2½ mile run; ½ mile walk
THURS:	rest and recover
FRI:	½ mile walk; 2½ mile run; ½ mile walk
SAT:	½ mile walk; 2¾ mile run; ½ mile walk
SUN:	rest and recover

WEEK SEVEN

MON:	½ mile walk; 2½ mile run; ½ mile walk
TUES:	rest and recover
WED:	½ mile walk; 2½ mile run; ½ mile walk
THURS:	rest and recover
FRI:	½ mile walk; 2½ mile run; ½ mile walk
SAT:	½ mile walk; 2¾ mile run; ½ mile walk
SUN:	rest and recover

WEEK EIGHT

MON:	½ mile walk; 2¾ mile run; ½ mile walk
TUES:	rest and recover

WED: ½ mile walk; 2¾ mile run; ½ mile walk

THURS: rest and recover

FRI: ½ mile walk; 2¾ mile run; ½ mile walk

SAT: ½ mile walk; 3 mile run; ½ mile walk

SUN: rest and recover

THE THIRD MONTH

WEEK NINE

MON: ½ mile walk; 3 mile run; ½ mile walk

TUES: rest and recover

WED: ½ mile walk; 3 mile run; ½ mile walk

THURS: rest and recover

FRI: ½ mile walk; 3 mile run; ½ mile walk

SAT: ½ mile walk; 3¼ mile run; ½ mile walk

SUN: rest and recover

WEEK TEN

MON: ½ mile walk; 3¼ mile run; ½ mile walk

TUES: rest and recover

WED: ½ mile walk; 3¼ mile run; ½ mile walk

THURS: rest and recover

FRI: ½ mile walk; 3¼ mile run; ½ mile walk

SAT: ½ mile walk; 3½ mile run; ½ mile walk

SUN: rest and recover

WEEK ELEVEN

MON: ½ mile walk; 3½ mile run; ½ mile walk

TUES: rest and recover

WED: ½ mile walk; 3½ mile run; ½ mile walk

THURS: rest and recover

FRI: ½ mile walk; 3½ mile run; ½ mile walk

SAT: ½ mile walk; 3¾ mile run; ½ mile walk

SUN: rest and recover

WEEK TWELVE: RACE WEEK

MON: ½ mile walk; 2 mile run

TUES: rest and recover

WED: ½ mile walk; 2 mile run

THURS: rest and recover

FRI: ½ mile walk; 1 mile run

SAT: Your first 5K race!

SUN: rest, recover, and celebrate

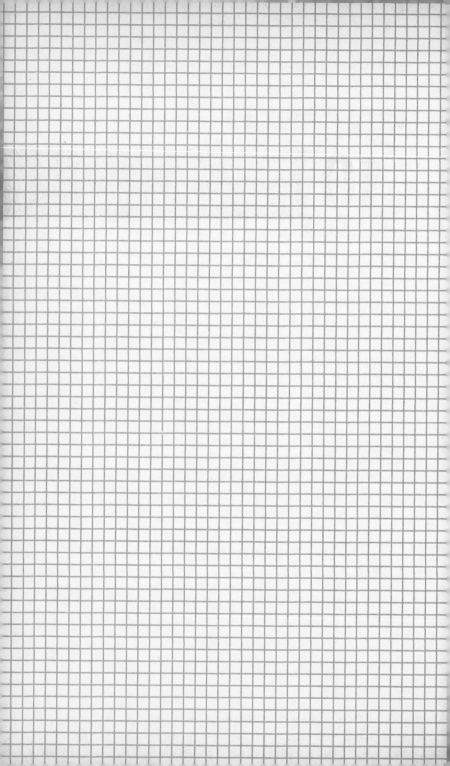

10 34-Minute Time-Goal Schedule

11-MINUTE PER MILE PACE

THE FIRST MONTH

WEEK ONE

MON: walk ½ mile to warm up; run ½ mile; walk ½ mile to cool down

TUES: rest and recover

WED: walk ½ mile to warm up; run ½ mile; walk ½ mile to cool down

THURS: rest and recover

FRI: walk ½ mile to warm up; run ½ mile; walk ½ mile to cool down

SAT: walk ½ mile to warm up; run ¾ mile; walk ½ mile to cool down

SUN: rest and recover

WEEK TWO

MON:	walk ½ mile to warm up; run ¾ mile; walk ½ mile to cool down
TUES:	rest and recover
WED:	walk ½ mile to warm up; run 1 mile; walk ½ mile to cool down
THURS:	rest and recover
FRI:	walk ½ mile to warm up; run 1 mile; walk ½ mile to cool down
SAT:	walk ½ mile to warm up; run 1¾ miles; walk ½ mile to cool down
SUN:	rest and recover

WEEK THREE

MON:	walk ½ mile to warm up; run 1¾ miles; ½ mile to cool down
TUES:	rest and recover
WED:	walk ½ mile to warm up; run 1¾ miles; ½ mile to cool down
THURS:	rest and recover
FRI:	walk ½ mile to warm up; run 1¾ miles; ½ mile to cool down
SAT:	walk ½ mile to warm up; run 2 miles; ½ mile to cool down
SUN:	rest and recover

WEEK FOUR

MON:	½ mile walk; 2 mile run; ½ mile walk
TUES:	rest and recover
WED:	½ mile walk; 2 mile run; ½ mile walk

THURS: rest and recover

FRI: ½ mile walk; 2 mile run; ½ mile walk

SAT: ½ mile walk; 2¼ mile run; ½ mile walk

SUN: rest and recover

WEEK FIVE

MON: ½ mile walk; 2¼ mile run; ½ mile walk

TUES: rest and recover

WED: ½ mile walk; 2 x ½ mile @ 5:30; ½ mile walk

THURS: rest and recover

FRI: ½ mile walk; 2¼ mile run; ½ mile walk

SAT: ½ mile walk; 2½ mile run; ½ mile walk

SUN: rest and recover

WEEK SIX

MON: ½ mile walk; 2½ mile run; ½ mile walk

TUES: rest and recover

WED: ½ mile walk; 3 x ½ mile @ 5:30; ½ mile walk

THURS: rest and recover

FRI: ½ mile walk; 2½ mile run; ½ mile walk

SAT: ½ mile walk; 2¾ mile run; ½ mile walk

SUN: rest and recover

WEEK SEVEN

MON: ½ mile walk; 2½ mile run; ½ mile walk

TUES: rest and recover

WED: ½ mile walk; 3 x ½ mile @ 5:30; ½ mile walk

THURS: rest and recover

FRI: ½ mile walk; 2½ mile run; ½ mile walk

SAT: ½ mile walk; 2¾ mile run; ½ mile walk

SUN: rest and recover

WEEK EIGHT

MON:	½ mile walk; 2¾ mile run; ½ mile walk
TUES:	rest and recover
WED:	½ mile walk; 4 x ½ mile @ 5:30; ½ mile walk
THURS:	rest and recover
FRI:	½ mile walk; 2¾ mile run; ½ mile walk
SAT:	½ mile walk; 3 mile run; ½ mile walk
SUN:	rest and recover

THE THIRD MONTH

WEEK NINE

MON:	½ mile walk; 3 mile run; ½ mile walk
TUES:	rest and recover
WED:	½ mile walk; 4 x ½ mile @ 5:30; ½ mile walk
THURS:	rest and recover
FRI:	½ mile walk; 3 mile run; ½ mile walk
SAT:	½ mile walk; 3¼ mile run; ½ mile walk
SUN:	rest and recover

WEEK TEN

MON:	½ mile walk; 3¼ mile run; ½ mile walk
TUES:	rest and recover
WED:	½ mile walk; 2 x 1 mile @ 11:00; ½ mile walk
THURS:	rest and recover
FRI:	½ mile walk; 3¼ mile run; ½ mile walk
SAT:	½ mile walk; 3½ mile run; ½ mile walk
SUN:	rest and recover

WEEK ELEVEN

MON:	½ mile walk; 3½ mile run; ½ mile walk
TUES:	rest and recover

WED:	½ mile walk; 2 x 1 mile @ 11:00; ½ mile walk
THURS:	rest and recover
FRI:	½ mile walk; 3½ mile run; ½ mile walk
SAT:	½ mile walk; 3¾ mile run; ½ mile walk
SUN:	rest and recover

WEEK TWELVE: RACE WEEK

MON:	½ mile walk; 2 mile run
TUES:	rest and recover
WED:	½ mile walk; 2 mile run
THURS:	rest and recover
FRI:	½ mile walk; 1 mile run
SAT:	Your first 5K race!
SUN:	rest, recover, and celebrate

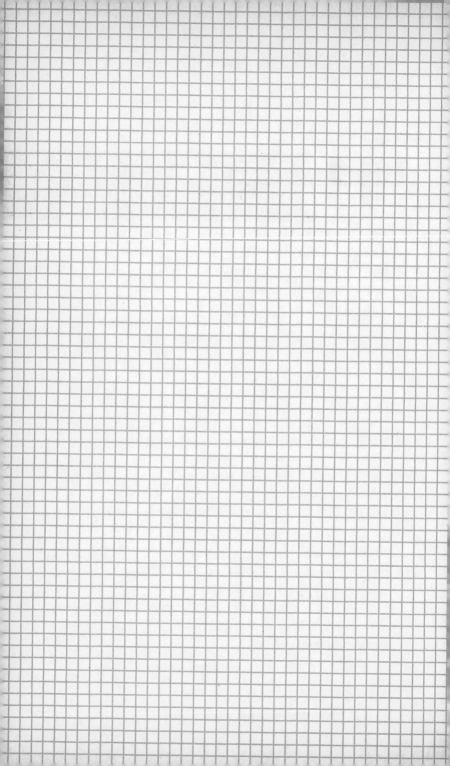

11 32-Minute Time-Goal Schedule

10:20-MINUTE PER MILE PACE

THE FIRST MONTH

WEEK ONE

MON: walk ½ mile to warm up; run ½ mile; walk ½ mile to cool down

TUES: rest and recover

WED: walk ½ mile to warm up; run ½ mile; walk ½ mile to cool down

THURS: rest and recover

FRI: walk ½ mile to warm up; run ½ mile; walk ½ mile to cool down

SAT: walk ½ mile to warm up; run ¾ mile; walk ½ mile to cool down

SUN: rest and recover

WEEK TWO

MON: walk ½ mile to warm up; run ¾ mile; walk ½ mile to cool down

TUES: rest and recover

WED: walk ½ mile to warm up; run 1 mile; walk ½ mile to cool down

THURS: rest and recover

FRI: walk ½ mile to warm up; run 1 mile; walk ½ mile to cool down

SAT: walk ½ mile to warm up; run 1¾ miles; walk ½ mile to cool down

SUN: rest and recover

WEEK THREE

MON: walk ½ mile to warm up; run 1¾ miles; ½ mile to cool down

TUES: rest and recover

WED: walk ½ mile to warm up; run 1¾ miles; ½ mile to cool down

THURS: rest and recover

FRI: walk ½ mile to warm up; run 1¾ miles; ½ mile to cool down

SAT: walk ½ mile to warm up; run 2 miles; ½ mile to cool down

SUN: rest and recover

WEEK FOUR

MON: ½ mile walk; 2 mile run; ½ mile walk

TUES: rest and recover

WED: ½ mile walk; 2 mile run; ½ mile walk

THURS: rest and recover

FRI: ½ mile walk; 2 mile run; ½ mile walk

SAT: ½ mile walk; 2¼ mile run; ½ mile walk

SUN: rest and recover

THE SECOND MONTH

WEEK FIVE

MON: ½ mile walk; 2¼ mile run; ½ mile walk

TUES: rest and recover

WED: ½ mile walk; 2 x ½ mile @ 5:10; ½ mile walk

THURS: rest and recover

FRI: ½ mile walk; 2¼ mile run; ½ mile walk

SAT: ½ mile walk; 2½ mile run; ½ mile walk

SUN: rest and recover

WEEK SIX

MON: ½ mile walk; 2½ mile run; ½ mile walk

TUES: rest and recover

WED: ½ mile walk; 3 x ½ mile @ 5:10; ½ mile walk

THURS: rest and recover

FRI: ½ mile walk; 2½ mile run; ½ mile walk

SAT: ½ mile walk; 2¾ mile run; ½ mile walk

SUN: rest and recover

WEEK SEVEN

MON: ½ mile walk; 2½ mile run; ½ mile walk

TUES: rest and recover

WED: ½ mile walk; 3 x ½ mile @ 5:10; ½ mile walk

THURS: rest and recover

FRI: ½ mile walk; 2½ mile run; ½ mile walk

SAT: ½ mile walk; 2¾ mile run; ½ mile walk

SUN: rest and recover

WEEK EIGHT

MON: ½ mile walk; 2¾ mile run; ½ mile walk

TUES: rest and recover

WED: ½ mile walk; 4 x ½ mile @ 5:10; ½ mile walk

THURS: rest and recover

FRI: ½ mile walk; 2¾ mile run; ½ mile walk

SAT: ½ mile walk; 3 mile run; ½ mile walk

SUN: rest and recover

THE THIRD MONTH

WEEK NINE

MON: ½ mile walk; 3 mile run; ½ mile walk

TUES: rest and recover

WED: ½ mile walk; 4 x ½ mile @ 5:10; ½ mile walk

THURS: rest and recover

FRI: ½ mile walk; 3 mile run; ½ mile walk

SAT: ½ mile walk; 3¼ mile run; ½ mile walk

SUN: rest and recover

WEEK TEN

MON: ½ mile walk; 3¼ mile run; ½ mile walk

TUES: rest and recover

WED: ½ mile walk; 2 x 1 mile @ 10:20; ½ mile walk

THURS: rest and recover

FRI: ½ mile walk; 3¼ mile run; ½ mile walk

SAT: ½ mile walk; 3½ mile run; ½ mile walk

SUN: rest and recover

WEEK ELEVEN

MON: ½ mile walk; 3½ mile run; ½ mile walk

TUES: rest and recover

WED:	½ mile walk; 2 x 1 mile @ 10:20; ½ mile walk
THURS:	rest and recover
FRI:	½ mile walk; 3½ mile run; ½ mile walk
SAT:	½ mile walk; 3¾ mile run; ½ mile walk
SUN:	rest and recover

WEEK TWELVE: RACE WEEK

MON:	½ mile walk; 2 mile run
TUES:	rest and recover
WED:	½ mile walk; 2 mile run
THURS:	rest and recover
FRI:	½ mile walk; 1 mile run
SAT:	Your first 5K race!
SUN:	rest, recover, and celebrate

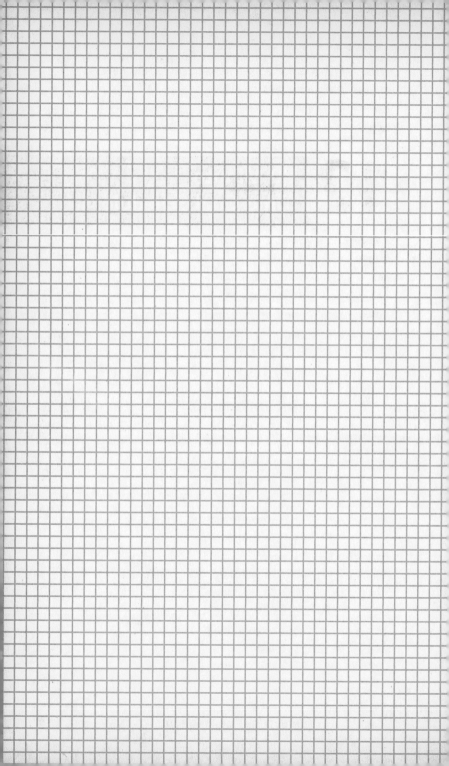

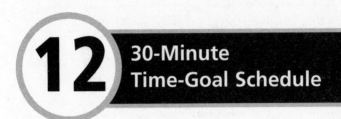

30-Minute Time-Goal Schedule

9:40-MINUTE PER MILE PACE

THE FIRST MONTH

WEEK ONE

MON: walk ½ mile to warm up; run ½ mile; walk ½ mile to cool down

TUES: rest and recover

WED: walk ½ mile to warm up; run ½ mile; walk ½ mile to cool down

THURS: rest and recover

FRI: walk ½ mile to warm up; run ½ mile; walk ½ mile to cool down

SAT: walk ½ mile to warm up; run ¾ mile; walk ½ mile to cool down

SUN: rest and recover

WEEK TWO

MON: walk ½ mile to warm up; run ¾ mile;
walk ½ mile to cool down

TUES: rest and recover

WED: walk ½ mile to warm up; run 1 mile;
walk ½ mile to cool down

THURS: rest and recover

FRI: walk ½ mile to warm up; run 1 mile;
walk ½ mile to cool down

SAT: walk ½ mile to warm up; run 1¾ miles;
½ mile to cool down

SUN: rest and recover

WEEK THREE

MON: walk ½ mile to warm up; run 1¾ miles;
½ mile to cool down

TUES: rest and recover

WED: walk ½ mile to warm up; run 1¾ miles;
½ mile to cool down

THURS: rest and recover

FRI: walk ½ mile to warm up; run 1¾ miles;
½ mile to cool down

SAT: walk ½ mile to warm up; run 2 miles;
½ mile to cool down

SUN: rest and recover

WEEK FOUR

MON: ½ mile walk; 2 mile run; ½ mile walk

TUES: rest and recover

WED: ½ mile walk; 2 mile run; ½ mile walk

THURS: rest and recover

FRI: ½ mile walk; 2 mile run; ½ mile walk

SAT: ½ mile walk; 2¼ mile run; ½ mile walk

SUN: rest and recover

WEEK FIVE

MON: ½ mile walk; 2¼ mile run; mile walk

TUES: rest and recover

WED: ½ mile walk; 2 x ½ mile @ 4:50; ½ mile walk

THURS: rest and recover

FRI: ½ mile walk; 2¼ mile run; ½ mile walk

SAT: ½ mile walk; 2½ mile run; ½ mile walk

SUN: rest and recover

THE SECOND MONTH

WEEK SIX

MON: ½ mile walk; 2½ mile run; ½ mile walk

TUES: rest and recover

WED: ½ mile walk; 3 x ½ mile @ 4:50; ½ mile walk

THURS: rest and recover

FRI: ½ mile walk; 2½ mile run; ½ mile walk

SAT: ½ mile walk; 2¾ mile run; ½ mile walk

SUN: rest and recover

WEEK SEVEN

MON: ½ mile walk; 2½ mile run; ½ mile walk

TUES: rest and recover

WED: ½ mile walk; 3 x ½ mile @ 4:50; ½ mile walk

THURS: rest and recover

FRI: ½ mile walk; 2½ mile run; ½ mile walk

SAT: ½ mile walk; 2¾ mile run; ½ mile walk

SUN: rest and recover

MON: ½ mile walk; 2¾ mile run; ½ mile walk

TUES: rest and recover

WED: ½ mile walk; 4 x ½ mile @ 4:50; ½ mile walk

THURS: rest and recover

FRI: ½ mile walk; 2¾ mile run; ½ mile walk

SAT: ½ mile walk; 3 mile run; ½ mile walk

SUN: rest and recover

THE THIRD MONTH

WEEK NINE

MON: ½ mile walk; 3 mile run; ½ mile walk

TUES: rest and recover

WED: ½ mile walk; 4 x ½ mile @ 4:50; ½ mile walk

THURS: rest and recover

FRI: ½ mile walk; 3 mile run; ½ mile walk

SAT: ½ mile walk; 3¼ mile run; ½ mile walk

SUN: rest and recover

WEEK TEN

MON: ½ mile walk; 3¼ mile run; ½ mile walk

TUES: rest and recover

WED: ½ mile walk; 2 x 1 mile @ 9:40; ½ mile walk

THURS: rest and recover

FRI: ½ mile walk; 3¼ mile run; ½ mile walk

SAT: ½ mile walk; 3½ mile run; ½ mile walk

SUN: rest and recover

WEEK ELEVEN

MON: ½ mile walk; 3½ mile run; ½ mile walk

TUES: rest and recover

WED: ½ mile walk; 2 x 1 mile @ 9:40; ½ mile walk

THURS: rest and recover

FRI: ½ mile walk; 3½ mile run; ½ mile walk

SAT: ½ mile walk; 3¾ mile run; ½ mile walk

SUN: rest and recover

WEEK TWELVE: RACE WEEK

MON: ½ mile walk; 2 mile run

TUES: rest and recover

WED: ½ mile walk; 2 mile run

THURS: rest and recover

FRI: ½ mile walk; 1 mile run

SAT: Your first 5K race!

SUN: rest, recover, and celebrate

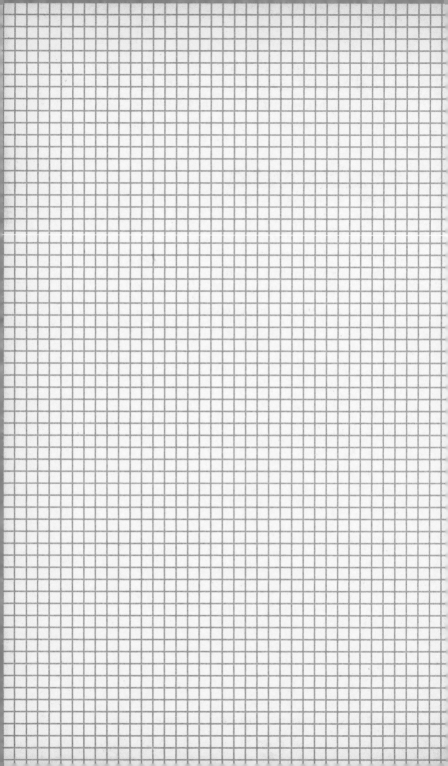

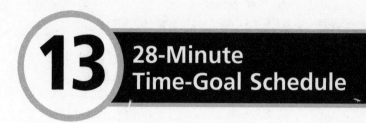

28-Minute Time-Goal Schedule

9-MINUTE PER MILE PACE

THE FIRST MONTH

WEEK ONE

MON:	walk ½ mile to warm up; run ½ mile; walk ½ mile to cool down
TUES:	rest and recover
WED:	walk ½ mile to warm up; run ½ mile; walk ½ mile to cool down
THURS:	rest and recover
FRI:	walk ½ mile to warm up; run ½ mile; walk ½ mile to cool down
SAT:	walk ½ mile to warm up, run ¾ mile; walk ½ mile to cool down
SUN:	rest and recover

WEEK TWO

MON: walk ½ mile to warm up; run ¾ mile;
walk ½ mile to cool down

TUES: rest and recover

WED: walk ½ mile to warm up; run 1 mile;
walk ½ mile to cool down

THURS: rest and recover

FRI: walk ½ mile to warm up; run 1 mile;
walk ½ mile to cool down

SAT: walk ½ mile to warm up; run 1¾ miles;
walk ½ mile to cool down

SUN: rest and recover

WEEK THREE

MON: walk ½ mile to warm up; run 1¾ miles;
½ mile to cool down

TUES: rest and recover

WED: walk ½ mile to warm up; run 1¾ miles;
½ mile to cool down

THURS: rest and recover

FRI: walk ½ mile to warm up; run 1¾ miles;
½ mile to cool down

SAT: walk ½ mile to warm up; run 2 miles;
½ mile to cool down

SUN: rest and recover

WEEK FOUR

MON: ½ mile walk; 2 mile run; ½ mile walk

TUES: rest and recover

WED: ½ mile walk; 2 mile run; ½ mile walk

THURS: rest and recover

FRI: ½ mile walk; 2 mile run; ½ mile walk

SAT: ½ mile walk; 2¼ mile run; ½ mile walk

SUN: rest and recover

THE SECOND MONTH

WEEK FIVE

MON: ½ mile walk; 2¼ mile run; ½ mile walk

TUES: rest and recover

WED: ½ mile walk; 2 x ½ mile @ 4:30; ½ mile walk

THURS: rest and recover

FRI: ½ mile walk; 2¼ mile run; ½ mile walk

SAT: ½ mile walk; 2½ mile run; ½ mile walk

SUN: rest and recover

WEEK SIX

MON: ½ mile walk; 2½ mile run; ½ mile walk

TUES: rest and recover

WED: ½ mile walk; 3 x ½ mile @ 4:30; ½ mile walk

THURS: rest and recover

FRI: ½ mile walk; 2½ mile run; ½ mile walk

SAT: ½ mile walk; 2¾ mile run; ½ mile walk

SUN: rest and recover

WEEK SEVEN

MON: ½ mile walk; 2½ mile run; ½ mile walk

TUES: rest and recover

WED: ½ mile walk; 3 x ½ mile @ 4:30; ½ mile walk

THURS: rest and recover

FRI: ½ mile walk; 2½ mile run; ½ mile walk

SAT: ½ mile walk; 2¾ mile run; ½ mile walk

SUN: rest and recover

WEEK EIGHT

MON: ½ mile walk; 2¾ mile run; ½ mile walk

TUES: rest and recover

WED: ½ mile walk; 4 x ½ mile @ 4:30; ½ mile walk

THURS: rest and recover

FRI: ½ mile walk; 2¾ mile run; ½ mile walk

SAT: ½ mile walk; 3 mile run; ½ mile walk

SUN: rest and recover

THE THIRD MONTH

WEEK NINE

MON: ½ mile walk; 3 mile run; ½ mile walk

TUES: rest and recover

WED: ½ mile walk; 4 x ½ mile @ 4:30; ½ mile walk

THURS: rest and recover

FRI: ½ mile walk; 3 mile run; ½ mile walk

SAT: ½ mile walk; 3¼ mile run; ½ mile walk

SUN: rest and recover

WEEK TEN

MON: ½ mile walk; 3¼ mile run; ½ mile walk

TUES: rest and recover

WED: ½ mile walk; 2 x 1 mile @ 9:00; ½ mile walk

THURS: rest and recover

FRI: ½ mile walk; 3¼ mile run; ½ mile walk

SAT: ½ mile walk; 3½ mile run; ½ mile walk

SUN: rest and recover

WEEK ELEVEN

MON: ½ mile walk; 3½ mile run; ½ mile walk

TUES: rest and recover

WED: ½ mile walk; 2 x 1 mile @ 9:00; ½ mile walk

THURS: rest and recover

FRI: ½ mile walk; 3½ mile run; ½ mile walk

SAT: ½ mile walk; 3¾ mile run; ½ mile walk

SUN: rest and recover

WEEK TWELVE: RACE WEEK

MON: ½ mile walk; 2 mile run

TUES: rest and recover

WED: ½ mile walk; 2 mile run

THURS: rest and recover

FRI: ½ mile walk; 1 mile run

SAT: Your first 5K race!

SUN: rest, recover, and celebrate

PART

4

YOUR FIRST 5K AND FUTURE RACES

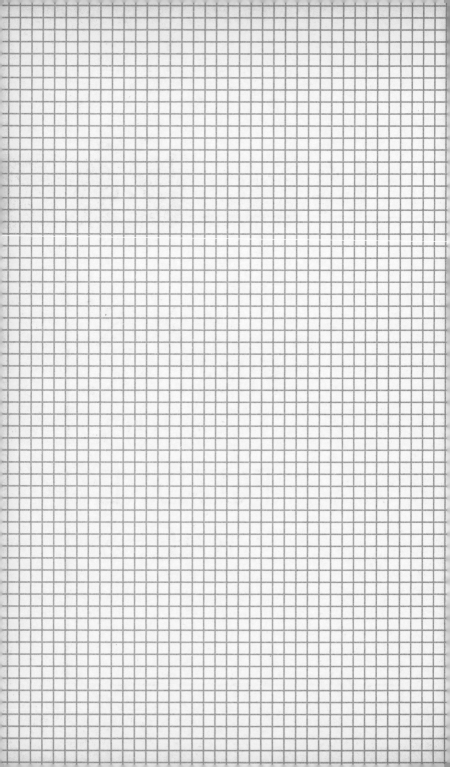

14 The Race

YOU'VE MADE IT through three months of training for your first 5K. You've built your endurance—from half a mile to where you can run more than the 5K distance without stopping—and you've rested and recovered well to make sure that you didn't overdo it. And if you followed one of the time-goal schedules, you've built up your strength to where you can run at race-goal pace with confidence.

Now comes the really fun stuff. Really. The race. You might feel butterflies in your stomach the day before or even the week before your first race (and if you don't feel nervous, great!), but the race experience will turn out to be a lot of fun. Trust me. There is something about testing yourself in a group of runners, going against the clock, and trying to get to the finish line that will prove to be one of the most rewarding and fun experiences in your life.

So the goal of this chapter is to make sure you are race ready: maybe a bit nervous, but full of anticipatory confidence for the race ahead. This will involve a state of mind that you develop at the beginning of race week, a checklist of things for you to do on race day (and the day before), and finally, strategies you'll employ during the race itself.

RACE-WEEK MIND-SET

EXACTLY ONE WEEK before your race, you should perform a "dry run." I don't mean that you should race a 5K in practice. The distance you'll cover will just be your normal, scheduled workout, but you'll approach it as though it were your race.

This means that starting the day before, you should be resting, eating well, drinking to make sure you aren't dehydrated; sleeping well; getting up in plenty of time to eat a small breakfast (if you think you need it); and wearing the shoes, shorts, and other stuff that you'll run the race in. In short, do a practice run of all the things you'll need to do the day before the race and on the actual race day.

This dry run serves two purposes:

1. It's a practice run for your race. You'll get used to what you will need to do, anticipate what might go wrong (say, if you eat something that upsets your stomach, you'll know not to eat that the day before or on race morning), and fill yourself with confidence for the same time next week.

2. It gets you focused on the race. When you run the race, you'll be in a different mental and emotional

state than you have been during the previous three months of training. During that time you were building endurance, speed, and confidence while anticipating the gradual increases you'd make in the weeks to come. Now, however, you are one week out from the race, and you need to shift into a different mode. You are no longer working toward a nebulous goal off in the distance, but something that is just one week away—and counting.

So how will the week before your race go? For starters, you should be getting more sleep. Try to go to bed at least a half hour earlier than you normally do and/or sleep in a half hour later (if this is possible with your schedule). Eat a few more carbs, but not too many. You don't need to stuff yourself to fuel up for the 5K, but you should feel like your leg muscles are full of muscle glycogen rather than depleted. This could simply mean having an extra half portion of carbohydrates once a day. For example, if your standard breakfast includes two pieces of toast, have three. Or if your standard dinner is a certain portion of spaghetti, have half a portion more. (Of course, if this makes you uncomfortable, don't do it.) You should also be drinking a bit more on these days. You can do this by simply adding a sixteen-ounce bottle of energy drink each day.

Also take time each day to spend five or ten minutes thinking about your race strategy (more in the box on page 116) and, in general, do things that relax you, rather than stress you out, when you're at work and at home. Finally review your training schedule to see how far you've come and to instill yourself with more confidence for race day.

Visualize Success

WHAT MENTAL METHODS can you use to get to the finish line of your first 5K on time? During the race you need to concentrate on your race strategy, as well as staying smooth and relaxed. But is there anything you can do, brainwise, in the days before the race to help you out on race day? Yes, there is. Something that competitive athletes in all sports use is a technique called visualization. Essentially what you are doing is "seeing your success." With your mind's eye, you picture the race developing the way you want it to.

For example: It's Wednesday evening before your first 5K, which will be run on Saturday. Dinner is over and you retreat to the den, where you have this book on your desk and some running posters up for motivation. You sit back in your easy chair. It is quiet. You close your eyes and picture this sequence:

1. You at the starting line in the middle of a huge crowd. Nervous, but in a good way. You're rested and ready, itching to begin.
2. The gun goes off. You remember your Starting-Gun Striders and work with the crowd, careful not to use too much energy and adrenaline at the start. That's a freshman mistake.
3. The crowd starts to thin out around the half-mile mark. You are on pace. Arms and shoulders loose. Head straight. Your breathing is controlled. There might even be a little smile on your face.

4. At the mile. Exact pace! You give yourself an inward thumbs-up and push on.
5. A few people pass you, and you pass others. You know your first race is not about beating other runners; it's about the only true race there is in the world—a race with yourself. And you know you can run to your potential.
6. The second mile is the mental one. You see yourself concentrating, focusing ahead, making a mental effort here as much as a physical one. You are keeping the pace and you are strong.
7. Two miles. Right on target again. But now you know that you need to push through some pain. You keep the pace steady. You don't even think about slowing down.
8. A half-mile out. You are tired and sweaty, but at the same time totally energized. The finish line is almost in sight.
9. There it is, the finish-line banner. Your first 5K finish is in view. You hold your form and push onward.
10. At the line you look at the clock. *Got it!* You have finished your first 5K in your goal time.

Then open your eyes and smile. Tomorrow night after dinner you'll do the same visualization. And you can't wait to see your victory again.

RACE-DAY (AND THE DAY BEFORE) CHECKLIST

HERE IS A checklist of things you need to do to prepare yourself for your first 5K, starting the day before the race:

1. Get out your racing gear: This means having your shoes, socks, shorts, shirt, hat, sports watch—everything you'll be wearing—laid out in your bedroom or den. With this done, you won't be nervous about it the night before—or, worse, racing around the house looking for this stuff on race-day morning.

2. If you have your race number already, put it with your other gear. You should register early for the race if possible to save race-morning anxiety. (For more on registration, see page 121.) Make sure you have four pins to attach your number to your shirt. (You do this at the corners, making sure your race number hangs midway down your rib cage, not across the chest, where it can impede your arm swing while you run.)

3. If you haven't registered yet, make sure you have the money for the entry fee ready for the morning.

4. Check your shoelaces. They should be firm and not frayed. If there are any doubts about the tensile strength of the laces, take them out and put in new ones. There are few things worse just before a race than tying your shoes and hearing a snap as a lace breaks.

5. Set the alarm clock. And then the one on your running watch. Having two alarms set prevents that middle-of-the-night fear that your alarm clock will

fail to go off and you'll miss the race. (You can also have a trusted running friend call you at a certain time in the morning and vice versa.)

6. If you'll be driving to the race, make sure you've got gas in the tank. You don't need to worry about this in the morning, either.

7. Double-check to make sure you know exactly how to get to the race site. Print out a map if you need one.

8. Pack extras, like a towel, fresh socks, a change of clothes and shoes for after the race (you don't want to wear your sweaty running clothes then), a bottle of water or energy drink, and a postrace snack, like an apple, banana, or bagel. If you wear contacts, bring along a spare pair, just in case.

9. If you'll be waking up extremely early for the race and you live with your family, you might want to kiss them good night and good morning before you go to bed—unless, of course, they'll be cheering you on at the big event.

10. On race morning, get up in plenty of time to be fully awake and get everything done. Even if your race is virtually next door, try the two-hour rule. Get up two hours before the starting time of the race and:

   a. Eat your light breakfast, making sure to drink two glasses of water.

   b. Take a quick shower. It helps you wake up and keeps nervous, prerace sweat from making you feel sticky.

   c. Put on your race clothes. If you feel like it, wear a light sweat suit or a pair of walking shorts over your running shorts; these will be more comfortable to drive in.

11. Leave home in time to get to the race about forty-five minutes before the start (if you haven't yet registered, make that an hour). Any less time and you'll feel nervous on the drive over, rushed to get your warm-up in, and tired from wasting energy on anxiety. Any more time, however, and you'll find yourself standing around getting impatient.

12. Warm up. Jog for ten minutes and then do some light stretching. Drink a cup or two of water, which should be provided by the race organizers at the starting area—or go back to your car and swig some from the water bottle you brought along. (You definitely don't want to be thirsty at the start of a race.)

13. About ten minutes before the start, position yourself near the starting line. Gradually work your way into the middle or back of the pack of runners. Don't line up near the front; you'll just get bumped and shoved at the start—or else you'll start much too fast and find yourself tired and slowing down early in the race.

14. Recheck your shoelaces. Double knot them if you haven't done so already.

15. Make sure all the pins on your race number are secure.

16. Put your sports watch in stopwatch mode.

17. Wait for the starting command. And start your watch at the gun or horn or whistle.

18. Begin running, not at the starting signal but when the runners in front of you start to move.

19. Pay attention to when you cross the actual starting line, and when you do, glance at your watch. Note how long it's taken you to get there. After the race,

you can subtract those seconds (or even minutes, if it's a really big race) to get a better idea of your actual time for the distance.

Registered and Ready

IT USED TO be that everyone registered on race-day morning, and there was a nervous crush of latecomers at the registration tables just before the gun. Then races added the option of letting runners mail in their registrations early and pick up their race numbers at a special "already registered" desk—but you had to mail your entry in a week before the race due to the time delays of snail mail. Nowadays most races have online registration that can be used up to the day before the race—and then you can pick up your number before the race.

The information you will be asked to provide is simple: your name, age, sex, address, and sometimes your running-club affiliation (if you have one). You sign at the bottom to testify that you consider yourself in race shape and not a health risk.

It is recommended that you register ahead of time, so there's less hassle before the race and no chance that you might miss the start, which has happened to most long-time runners at least once.

STRATEGIC RACE COMMAND

THE 5K MAY be only 3.1 miles long,, but you still need to have a well thought-out race strategy in your head when you're standing on the starting line, preferably one you've been contemplating for weeks or more.

The most common mistake first-time runners make in the 5K is that when the gun goes off, they take off. Running way too fast for their training and fitness, they're dead on their feet by the time they reach the half-mile mark—shuffling, walking, or simply stopping in exhaustion and dropping out.

This won't happen if you've planned out your race strategy ahead of time. There are several possible strategies to choose from for a 5K.

Even Pacer

An even-pacer strategy simply means that you will try to run each of your three miles at the same pace.

If you're following the Survivor Schedule, you should use this strategy, since it prevents the buildup of lactic acid, the waste product of exercise that makes your legs burn and feel heavy. Lactic acid production is exacerbated by sudden shifts in race pace. Running at a steady pace also keeps your breathing easy and controlled.

If you're running a time-goal schedule, run as close to the exact race pace you've set for yourself as possible. (You'll be able to check your pace at each mile—in any well-organized race, there will be a mile marker and either a digital clock or a person reading off your time at that point—called your split time—as you pass.) For example, if you are aiming for a thirty-four-minute 5K, and you have gone through the training program for it in this book, then you'll be trying to run each mile in eleven minutes flat. Don't worry if the first mile passes in 11:03 or 11:06 or so. A steady pace in the second mile should make up the time difference (most of that time deficit might be due to the crowds at the start). Be sure to stay strong and steady, and resist the temptation to pick up the pace; stay confident that your even-pacer strategy will get you to the finish line on time.

Seconds Strategy

The even-pacer strategy should be used by complete beginners and all those who have gotten through their training programs without a hitch and have confidence in their ability to run. But what do you do if you feel just a little off? Say, the last few weeks were interrupted by work or family obligations, you've missed some important workouts, and you're just not confident of holding a steady pace.

Well, you can try for seconds. With this strategy, you'll work harder during the second mile—the hardest mile of the race in general—after easing into the race in the first mile. Then try to hold steady for the last mile. Basically you won't be tied to exact times for the miles. Your pace for a thirty-four-minute 5K might look like something like this: 11:12 (first mile), 10:50 (second mile), 10:58 (third mile).

With this strategy, you play it safe by starting with a conservative first mile. In the second mile you get serious and run hard, counting on the easy first mile—and the late-race excitement—to give you enough energy to hang on in mile three.

The Last-Gasp Strategy

A racing mistake turned into a strategy that still has benefits, the last gasp is almost self-explanatory: You run fairly easy for the first two miles, and then push it hard for the last mile, in a last gasp to get to the finish line. This strategy can work if you are slow to adjust to race pace at the start and a little wary of running out of gas if you compensate too quickly. You're putting all your racing eggs in one basket—the last mile—and your mile splits could look something like this: 11:08, 11:07; 10:45.

POST-RACE RECOVERY

ONCE YOU'VE FINISHED your 5K, you might think that the work is over, but it's not quite. You still have to recover from your first race. Simply walking to your car and driving home is no way to recover (or to enjoy the postrace festivities). It's far better to follow a postrace procedure that will ensure that when you wake up the next morning, your running career is still humming along smoothly.

To do this, follow these simple postrace steps:

1. **Keep moving:** The temptation once you cross the line will be to stop and sit. Walking away from the finish and continuing to walk for a while will do wonders for your postrace recovery.
2. **Drink:** Replenish yourself with the sports drink offered at the finish and then later from the bottle that you brought along.
3. **Jog a little:** Do about a half-mile at a very slow jog around the parking lot. This will flush the lactic acid and other waste products out of your legs.
4. **Eat an apple, a banana, or a bagel with peanut butter:** You need to fuel those muscles after your race, preferably within twenty minutes of your fin-

ish. This is when the muscles are more receptive to storing glycogen.

5. **Change into those fresh clothes that you brought along:** It's quite uncomfortable to have to hang around after a race, and then drive home, in sweaty running clothes.

15 What Next?

WHAT DO YOU do after this program is over, and you're sitting in the den with your race T-shirt on, your finisher's medal around your neck, considering opening a giant bag of chips? After all, you did it, right?

This moment will be a crucial one in your running life. You need to ask yourself a serious question: Did you take part in the program to simply complete a 5K and be done with it, moving on to bowling, Ping-Pong, or seven-card stud?

Or do you really want to be a runner?

If you've read this book, followed this program, and completed your first 5K, then I sincerely hope that you will look long and hard at the second option.

There are many forks that you can now take on the running path. Here are some that you might consider.

MAINTAIN

Maintaining simply means keeping up with the tenets you've learned in this program. Continue the daily runs—say, the ones in weeks ten and eleven—and use them as your guide for the next three, six, or twelve months. This will ensure that you keep running and are comfortable doing it

Along the way, you can jump into another 5K—or two, or three—to keep some variety and focus in your training. Then, when you're ready, you could consider one of the other options.

GET FASTER

If you want to progress in your running—and most runners do—you have two options: Run farther or run faster. The second option is your simplest bet right after completing the program the first time around. Simply rest a week, then start on a more ambitious program, say, going from the Survivor Schedule to the 34-Minute Schedule or from the 34-Minute Schedule to the 32-Minute Schedule. It's best to jump up only one schedule at a time. This will ensure that you don't burn out, get injured from suddenly trying to run too fast, and set yourself up for a major disappointment on your next race day (which will put negative thoughts about running into your head and quite possibly end your running career before it really gets started).

Because the next step is . . .

MOVE UP TO THE 10K AND THE HALF MARATHON

THE 10K IS twice the distance of the 5K: 10 kilometers; 6.2 miles. But it's more than twice as hard to train for. That's because you need more time to prepare—preferably another month, if you're serious about the distance. The endurance runs will be longer: 8 miles, 10 miles, even 12 miles. And the strength runs will be more demanding: 6 × 800 or 3 × 1 mile or 2 × 2 miles, for starters. And you'll need to run an extra day per week—five days, not four.

The half marathon is roughly 21.1 kilometers, approximately 13.1 miles—literally, half the distance of a marathon. While considered a serious challenge by many runners, it's a seemingly more approachable race than the marathon. It, too requires a different training regime.

You should educate yourself on these processes, either through a book or a local coach or both. Preferably both.

If you do decide to move up, don't forget the basic training tenets of this book along the way: Workouts should be increased in length and intensity very gradually, taking time for rest and recovery. And that your eventual race day should be treated with respect, which means that a taper (a backing-off, sharpening-up period) is in order, maybe more than one week's worth of rest and readiness.

THE MARATHON

MANY RUNNERS CONSIDER this the ultimate test: 26.2 miles, the longest standard road-race distance and the longest Olympic running event. What can I say? It's tough. You'll need to work hard, devote four to six months (or more) to training, and use knowledge from books, training programs, fellow runners, and maybe a coach, to make it every step of the way.

It is something that you, standing here now with this book in your hand, hopefully just after you've completed your first 5K, may decide to shoot for down the line. Give yourself a long-term running goal of two to three years or more. Every marathon except the Boston Marathon is open to any runner, regardless of your speed (though many major marathons like Chicago sell out of all their entry places early or use a lottery system like New York). So getting into some marathon is not likely to be a problem.

Training for it will be a challenge. I have written a simple, basic marathon training book, *4 Months to a 4-Hour Marathon,* that's sort of like the marathon-training version of *3 Months to Your First 5K.* I highly recommend it and/or other resources (other books, getting a coach, joining a running club, etc.) if you're considering a marathon in your future.

Resources

ONE OF MY favorite running resources is a magazine I have been associated with for almost twenty years—*Runner's World*. The U.S. edition has more than 600,000 subscribers, and *RW* now produces several distinct editions worldwide, including in the United Kingdom, Germany, South Africa, Italy, and Australia/New Zealand. *RW* can be found on any newsstand, or you can save money by getting a subscription. Its content is a modern mix of nutrition, training, gear, and lifestyle—plus top-notch features like travel stories or profiles of great runners (or runners whose stories are great).

Running Times magazine also covers the running world, but with a slant that's more toward the seasoned runner. The stories and training articles often assume a certain knowledge of the sport on the reader's part. There's more extensive race coverage than in *Runner's World*, in keeping with the slant toward the experienced runner.

Marathon and Beyond is a magazine that features training articles and marathon stories by some well-known writers and runners, but also by many everyday Janes and Joes.

Runner's World's website—www.runnersworld.com—is a great resource for what's happening in the daily world of running. The website is essentially a daily newspaper for the sport—it runs Monday through Friday and contains many links to *RW* training stories and features.

For the running obsessed, www.letsrun.com offers links seven days a week to news stories about running. Its message board is famous or infamous, depending on your perspective; there's a lot of expertise on display and a lot of very strongly expressed opinions as well. For an online atmosphere that's more tolerant of the beginner—and a place to log your workouts, ask for expert and friendly advice, and meet runners from around the world (and probably in your hometown)— try www.therunninglog.com.

Index

A
Achilles tendon, sore, 73
afternoon runs, 38
alcohol, 47
anxiety, 6

B
beer, 47
benefits of running, 5
black toenails, 72–73
Boston Marathon, 130
Boulder Running Company, 16
bras
    for heat, 28
    running, 21–22

C
calf stretch, 64–65
carbohydrates, 42, 115
charity, running for, 8–9
checklist, pre-race, 118–21
chondromalacia patellae
    (runner's knee), 72
cold tolerance, 26
cold weather gear, 25

D
depression, 6
distance
    5K length, reasons for, 11
    increasing, 128
    timing, 120–21
downhill grades, 71
dry run, 114–15

E
endurance run, 59
energy bars, 45–46
energy drinks, 29
evening runs, 39
even pacer strategy, 122–23

F
fat, 43
first race
    checklist, 118–21
    race-week mind-set, 114–15
    visualize success, 116–17
4 Months to a 4-Hour Marathon,
    130
fun in running, stages of, 7–8

G
gloves, 27
glycogen, 115, 125
Gore-Tex–type fiber, 25
   jacket, 27
grass fields, 35

H
half marathon, 129
hamstring stretch, 65–66
hat, running, 25
heat
   clothing for, 28
   running in, 28–29
hiking paths, 33
hot spots, 71–72
hydration, 29, 115, 124

I
ice, muscles and, 70
Iliotibial band. *See* IT band
injuries, 69–74
   prevention tips, 69–71
   types of, dealing with, 71–74
   see also individual injuries
IT band
   strain, 74
   stretch, 67

J
jackets, 27

L
lactic acid production, 122
last-gasp strategy, 123–24
late-morning runs, 37
letsrun.com, 132
lifestyle, running, 57
logbooks, 58
lower back stretch, 66
lunchtime runs, 37–38

M
maintaining, 128
marathon, 129–30
Marathon and Beyond magazine,
   131
meal plan, 43–47
morning runs, 36–37
motivation, 76–77
Muhrcke, Gary, 19–20
muscles
   glycogen and, 115, 125
   ice for soothing, 70
   lactic acid production and, 122
   strains, 71

N
night runs, 39
number, race, 118, 120
nutrition, 41–47
   alcohol, 47
   carbohydrates, 42
   energy bars, 45–46
   fat, 43
   meal plan, 43–44
   peanut butter, 43
   post race, 124–25
   protein, 42
   race day and, 119
   race week and, 115
   snacks, 45
   sports drinks, 46–47

P
peanut butter, 43
physical fitness, 5–6
Plaatjes, Mark, 16
post-race recovery, 124–25
protein, 42

Q
quadriceps stretch, 65

R

rain, 23–24
rain gear, 23
recovery run, 60–61
registration, 118, 121
roads, 33–34
runner's knee (chondromalacia
    patellae), 72
Runner's World, 131, 132
Runner Times magazine, 131
running form, 51–56
    breathing, 54
    first steps, 55–56
    Pride of Going Farther, 56–57
runninglog.com, 132

S

sciatica, 74
seconds strategy, 123
shin splints, 73–74
shirts, 22
    long-sleeved, 25
    T-shirts, 28
shoes, 15–20
    black toenails and, 72–73
    buying, 16–20
    drying, 24
    employee verification, 19
    hot spots and, 71–72
    injury prevention and, 70
    shoelaces, checking on race
        day, 118, 120
shorts, 22
sidewalks, 34
sleep, 115, 118–19
slide-off effect, 6
snacks, 45
snow, 23
socks, 20
soleus stretch, 66
speed, increasing, 128

Spence, Steve, 37
sports drinks, 46–47
starting-gun strider, 61
strategy, 121–24
    even pacer, 122–23
    last-gasp, 123–24
    seconds, 123
    thinking about, before race, 115
strength run, 60
stress, 6
stretching, 63–67
    to avoid injuries, 70
    calf stretch, 64–65
    hamstring stretch, 65–66
    IT band stretch, 67
    lower back stretch, 66
    quadriceps stretch, 65
    soleus stretch, 66
    time spent on, 63
    total back stretch, 67
    warming up, 64, 120
success, visualizing, 116–17
sunglasses, 22
sunscreen, 28
Super Runners Shops, 19–20
surfaces, running, 31–35
    downhill grades, 71
    grass fields, 35
    injury prevention and, 71
    roads, 33–34
    running trails vs. hiking
        paths, 33
    sidewalks, 34
    tracks, 32
    trails, 33
    treadmills, 34–35
survivor schedule, 76, 81–85,
    122, 128
Susan G. Komen Breast Cancer
    Foundation Race for the
    Cure, 8

T

10K race, 129
three- month time frame, reasons for, 9–10
tights, running, 27–28
time-goal schedules, 77–78, 87–91
   maintaining, 128
   during race, 122
   34-minute, 87–91
   32-minute, 93–97
   30-minute, 99–103
   28-minute, 105–9
time of day to run, 36–39
   afternoon, 38
   evening, 39
   late morning, 37
   lunchtime, 37–38
   morning, 36–37
   night, 39
timing, 120–21
total back stretch, 67
tracks, 32
trails, running, 33

training program, 57–61
   endurance run, 59
   logbooks, 58
   recovery run, 60–61
   starting-gun strider, 61
   strength run, 60
   walks, 59–60
training schedules, 76–79
   abbreviations used in, 79
   basic finisher (survivor), 76, 81–85
   illness and, 79
   motivation and, 76–77
   see also time-goal schedules
treadmills, 34–35

W

walks, 59–60
warming up, 64, 120
watch, sports, 20–21, 120
weight room, 7
well-being, 6–7
wine, 47